How to feed
your whole
family a healthy,
balanced diet

Acknowledgements

I'd like to thank the following people for passing on tips and recipes and sharing their knowledge and expertise. They are: housewives of the 1950s and 60s; Jean Hack, Barbara Holcombe, Irene Rutman, Doreen Gould, June Greenland, Daphne Croucher and Norah Pearce; also Tim Hack, Claire Orencas, Carole Moore and Sarah Todd – and last but not least my three children, Oliver, Billy and Eleanor who eat everything up and make it all worthwhile.

howto**books**
Please send for a free copy of the latest catalogue:
How To Books
Spring Hill House, Spring Hill Road,
Begbroke, Oxford OX5 1RX, United Kingdom
info@howtobooks.co.uk
www.howtobooks.co.uk

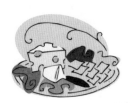
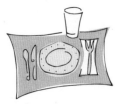
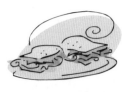

How to feed your whole family a healthy, balanced diet

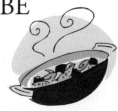

with very little money
and hardly any time,
even if you have a tiny
kitchen, only three
saucepans (one with an
ill-fitting lid) and no fancy
gadgets – unless you count
the garlic crusher…

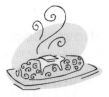

**Simple, wholesome and
nutritious recipes for family meals**

GILL HOLCOMBE

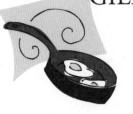
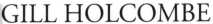

howtobooks

Published by Spring Hill

Spring Hill is an imprint of
How To Books Ltd
Spring Hill House, Spring Hill Road
Begbroke, Oxford OX5 1RX. United Kingdom.
Tel: (01865) 375794 Fax: (01865) 379162
info@howtobooks.co.uk
www.howtobooks.co.uk

British Library Cataloguing in Publication Data.
A catalogue record for this book is available
from the British Library.

First edition 2007
Reprinted 2008 (five times)

ISBN: 978 1 905862 15 3

Cover design by Baseline Arts Ltd
Produced for Spring Hill Books by Deer Park Productions, Tavistock
Typeset by Baseline Arts Ltd
Printed and bound by Bell & Bain Ltd, Glasgow

Contents

INTRODUCTION / 1
Where did we go wrong? / 1
The stumbling blocks...
what puts you off? / 7
A word about weight loss / 10
Everyday essentials / 11
Notes on preparing vegetables / 16

1 WAKE UP TO BREAKFAST / 21
Everyday breakfasts / 22
Weekend breakfasts / 28

2 LITTLE GEMS AND TOUGH
   COOKIES / 31
Fussy Eaters / 32
Packed Lunches / 36

3 MAKE DINNER, NOT EXCUSES / 43
Main recipes:
Shepherd's Pie / 44
Moussaka / 45
Chilli Con Carne / 47
Hamburgers / 49
Rissoles / 50
Chicken Nuggets / 52
Chicken Curry / 54
Mexican Chicken / 55
Chicken & Ham Pasta Bake / 57
Sweet & Sour Chicken / 58
Toad in the Hole / 60
Cider Sausages / 61
Sausage Rolls / 63
Sweet Apple & Apricot Pork / 65
Ginger Beer Pork / 66

Spicy Pork Meatballs / 66
Steak & Kidney Pudding / 68
Beef Stroganoff / 70
Lancashire Hot Pot / 71
Chicken Liver Risotto / 74
Tuna Lasagne / 77
Sweet & Spicy Prawns / 78
Kedgeree / 79
Fishcakes / 81
Stuffed Peppers / 83
Stuffed Mushrooms / 84
Veggie Burgers / 85
Aubergine Lasagne / 87
Lentil Moussaka / 88
Rice Salad / 90
Nut-free Nut Roast / 92
Pizza / 93
Baked Potato Pizzas / 96
Cheese & Onion Tomatoes / 97
DIY Pasta Sauce / 99
Ratatouille / 101

Recipes in brief:
Beef & Cheese Crumble / 51
Chicken in Cream & Mushroom Sauce / 59
Chicken Goujons / 59
Pork in Plum Sauce / 67
Greek-style Pork / 67
Kebabs / 72
Medallions of Lamb in Red Wine / 73
Liver in Black Bean Sauce / 75
Mixed Grill / 76
Spicy Liver & Pork Meatballs / 76
Fish Pie / 82
Grilled Sardines / 82

4 QUICK FIXES / 105
Quorn Stir Fry / 106
Pacific Pie / 107
Noodles / 108
More Noodles / 109
Bacon Cakes / 110
Devilled Kidneys / 111
One Step Pasta / 112
Instant Corned Beef Hash / 112
Prawn & Egg Pie / 113
Fish Finger Pie / 114
Smoked Salmon Tagliatelle / 115
Fastest-ever Fishcakes / 116
Things on Toast / 117

5 THE JOY OF SOUP / 119
Orange Squash / 120
Slug & Celery / 121
Watercress / 122
Stinging Nettle / 123
Sweet Potato / 124
Lentil & Vegetable / 125
Spicy Bean / 126
Tomato & Red Lentil / 127
Minestrone / 128
Smoked Mackerel Chowder / 130
Borsht / 131
Chicken / 132
Scotch Broth / 134
Cool Cucumber / 136
Hot or Cold Leek & Potato / 137

6 JOIN THE PUDDING CLUB / 141
Main recipes:
Cherry Cheesecake / 143
Lemon Cheesecake / 144
Cheshire Tart / 145

Baked Apples / 147
Rhubarb Crumble / 148
Poor Man's Apple Pie / 149
Jimmy Young Trifle / 150
Bread & Butter Pudding / 151
Raspberry Ice-Cream / 152
Chocolate Mousse / 153
Treacle Tart / 154
Tiramisu / 155
Fruit Fool / 156
Spotted Dick / 157

Recipes in brief:
Strawberry Meringues / 159
Orange Cups / 159
Baked Banana Custard / 159
Fruit Jelly / 159

7 CANT COOK? DONT COOK! / 161

8 LET THEM EAT CAKE / 165
Cooking with children:
Easy Cheesy Biscuits / 171
Cheese & Courgette Scones / 172
Jam Tarts / 173
Chocolate Rice Krispie Cakes / 174
Cornflake Cakes / 175
Fairy Cakes / 175
Gingerbread Men / 177
Sweetloaf / 178
Treacle Crunches / 180
Chocolate Chip Cookies / 180

Wholesome cakes:
Carrot Cake / 182
Bran Loaf / 183
Rock Buns / 184

Ginger Cake / 185
Banana Cake / 186
All-in-One Apple Cake / 187
Bread Pudding / 188
Flapjacks / 189
Seed Cake / 190
Plum Cake / 191
Apricot & Almond Muffins / 192
Muesli Muffins / 194
Pumpkin Muffins / 195

Special cakes:
Swiss Roll / 196
Caterpillar Cake / 199
Chocolate Yule Log / 200
Layer Cake / 201
Honey, Lemon & Yoghurt Cake / 202
The Ultimate Chocolate Cake / 203
Chocolate Caramel Cakes / 205

9 NOT ONLY BUT ALSO /209
Quick Brown Bread / 209
Soda Bread / 210
Garlic Bread / 212
Chicken Liver Pate / 213
Kipper Pate / 214
Guacamole / 214
Hummus / 215
Roasted Nuts / 216
Mayonnaise / 216
Potato Salad / 217
Hash Browns / 218
Hot Cross Buns / 219
Honeycomb / 222
Ginger Beer / 222
Toffee Apples / 224
Chutney / 226

Soft Fruit Spread / 227
Grapefruit Curd / 228
Figgy Pudding / 229
Fudge / 231

10 WEEKLY MENU PLANNING / 235
Chilli Con Carne & Rice / 239
Chilli & Chips / 239
Veggie Burgers & Potato Wedges / 240
Chinese Chicken Stir Fry / 241
Frankfurters & DIY Pasta Sauce / 241
Roast Chicken / 242
Chicken & Leek Casserole / 243
Bubble, Bangers & Beans / 244
Kedgeree / 245
Cheese & Spinach Omelette / 245
Boiled Bacon & Roasted Vegetables / 247
Vegetable Tortilla / 249
Pork Meatballs, Tagliatelli & Tomato
    Sauce / 250
Stuffed Peppers / 250
Pacific Pie / 250
Liver, Bacon & Onions / 252
Tomato & Red Lentil Soup / 253
Salmon & Tomato Pasta Bake / 253
Pork Ribs, Sausages & Rice / 253
Bread Roll Pizzas / 254
Corned Beef Hash / 256
Fish Finger Pie / 257
Spaghetti Bolognese / 257
Curried Nut Roast / 258
Gammon Steaks, Egg &
    Homemade
    Chips / 259
Index / 261

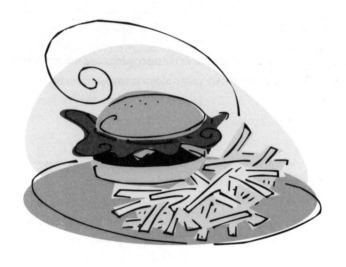

"Don't dig your grave
with your own knife and fork."

Old English proverb

Introduction

WHERE DID WE GO WRONG?

Have you ever spent a small fortune in the supermarket and still struggled to put a decent meal together? Are your children always complaining they're hungry even though they eat constantly? Do you own a set of expensive saucepans or have a kitchen full of gadgets you never use? Would you like to cook more and eat together as a family if only you had the time?

Time, or lack of it, is probably the reason most people give for not cooking, but less than 40 years ago practically everyone cooked at least one proper meal from scratch every day, even though very few people owned a fridge, let alone all the other labour-saving devices we take for granted today. Maybe we do have more commitments in some areas of our lives than previous generations, but when it comes to food, not only do we have a much greater variety to choose from, we also have 24-hour supermarkets, internet shopping, home deliveries, endless cookery programmes on TV, recipe books galore and microwave ovens that sell for smaller sums of money than you'd spend on a family meal in a fast food outlet.

To hear some people talk you'd think no one had ever been busy until about 1985, but no matter where you live or what your circumstances are, the truth is you can put a balanced meal together in less time that it takes to dial up a pizza and wait for it to be delivered (cold, usually) to your door. Nobody should have to rely on takeaways and ready meals, let alone feed them to their children, on a regular basis.

If recent reports are to be believed, there must be more cookery books gathering dust in designer kitchens in this country than there are people who actually cook anything. But having said that, it's simply not true that hardly anybody cooks from scratch either; lots of people combine a career with parenthood and still manage to produce decent food every day.

So apart from the old argument about having no time, what, exactly, is putting people off? Are they really too busy and important to roll their sleeves up and make a simple meal – or are they just lazy? Perhaps they don't care about the food they eat or they don't know where to start. Can there be anyone who doesn't realise how much better proper home-cooked food tastes than the mass-produced, cook-chill alternative? And that by preparing your food at home, your worst nightmares about what might have got into it by mistake – never mind what some people deliberately do to the food in factories for their own amusement – don't come into it? (Everyone's heard stories, and you must wonder sometimes, even if you've never had a bad experience yourself.)

Some of the blame must surely go to the manufacturers of convenience foods for making us believe that what they produce – so beautifully packaged and presented and cleverly advertised – is *good food,* and that by eating it we're making our lives easier. I bet there are hundreds of thousands of people who don't realise they could make far better shepherd's pie or lasagne themselves, just by following a very simple recipe – and why would they? So seductive are some of the TV commercials, you could be forgiven for thinking it's a privilege to be allowed inside the store to spend your money in the first place.

But make no mistake, no one's doing you any favours, least of all the major stores with their gorgeous displays, catchy slogans and phoney 'two for the price of one' deals. Not long ago I tried a 'cod goujon' from one of our biggest and best-loved stores at a friend's house. Biting into it I was horrified to discover it wasn't even a proper fish fillet, but a mishmash of whatever goes into the cheapest, low grade fish fingers. The only difference being that this 'goujon' wasn't shaped like a regular fish finger, presumably to give the impression that it was a superior product. Maybe the manufacturer wasn't committing any breach of the law (because the ingredients would have been hidden away in tiny writing on the packaging) but people in a hurry tend to grab whatever looks good and place their trust in the brand name, without stopping to study the small print, or even really knowing what they're looking for.

This isn't just food, this is inferior food. All they have to do is apply the current buzz words to everything, then sit back and wait for us to fall for it. I'm thinking of the 'organic' mash I came across in the same store recently, which costs more than a 10 lb sack of potatoes from a greengrocer. So what if it was 'organic'? I'd rather cook a few potatoes myself than spend £2 on one portion of mashed potatoes, which, looking at the label, is actually 82 per cent potato and 10 per cent fat. And, on the evidence of a friend who's actually eaten the organic mash, 'it doesn't really taste right', so no surprises there.

The funny thing about convenience food – at least it would be funny if we weren't the fattest nation in Europe and getting bigger all the time – is it's not even that convenient. Once you've removed the packaging, read the instructions, pierced the film lid (or not), waited, taken the tray out halfway through the cooking time to stir the food, waited again, let it stand for two minutes, scalded yourself on the steam, searched in vain for a piece of meat amongst the gunk, wolfed the lot in four minutes flat and wondered what else there is to eat because you're still hungry, it might occur to you that the little bit of effort you saved by not cooking your own dinner wasn't really justified by the end result. And the same can be said about so-called fast food, as anyone who has ever been served a burger at the counter in a fast food restaurant, then waited at the table (dirty, usually) for the fries to be brought over ten minutes later, will know.

The other food myth that often gets repeated is that the unhealthiest foods are necessarily the least expensive, and that some people, especially families on very low incomes, only resort to eating them because they have no choice. But this is nonsense. A week's worth of good quality meat and fish with lots of potatoes, rice, pasta, vegetables, fruit and other whole foods costs no more than the same amount of cheap chicken, burgers, pies, reconstituted potatoes, instant microwave meals and fizzy drinks.

I know cooking isn't everyone's idea of fun, and some people through no fault of their own are never going to enjoy it, which is why this book isn't about learning to cook complicated meals that take hours to prepare and only minutes for your kids to reject. You don't have to like cooking; you don't have to be a great cook, or even a particularly good one. You don't have to go shopping more often than you want to, or spend more money than you can afford. There's nothing here that you can't buy from any of the big supermarkets – assuming that's where you do your shopping because, like me, you're not lucky enough to have anything better where you live – and no expensive ingredients with unfamiliar names. Some of the recipes can be thrown together in minutes and a few don't involve any cooking at all. They all contain a certain amount of fat, sugar and salt, but nowhere near as much as you'd find in commercially prepared food – and at least the nutrients are there as well.

There seems to be a list of so-called super foods for everything and everybody these days; pregnancy, the menopause... I even came across a series of articles in one parenting magazine under what I thought was the very bad taste headline: 'Cancer-proof Your Kids'. One minute I'm reading about how I should be eating more purple food; the next week it's green, then orange and yellow. There's The Bikini Diet, The Sunset Beach Diet, The GMI Diet, The F-Plan Diet, low-fat-high-carb diets, high-fat-low-carb diets, and everything in between. Are we meant to be eating more, or *less* dairy right now? Is wheat an excellent source of fibre and slow-release carbohydrates, good for sustaining our energy levels – or a totally unnecessary food that many people have some kind of intolerance to? What should we be eating to be sure we're getting enough zinc? Is it a magnesium or potassium deficiency that causes sugar cravings? Sometimes, when you only want to know *what* is good for you, rather than *why,* it's too much information.

And yet, despite all this food knowledge, there are still people who think we need sugar for energy (not necessarily; we get energy from all our food), that diet colas are better than those containing sugar when they're potentially worse (because of the chemicals in artificial sweeteners), or who, when asked to name a typical English food say 'quiche'. I recently read that thousands of primary school children don't know where eggs come from, which is probably not surprising if it's also true – as yet another recent survey claims – that one-fifth of adults don't know which animals sausages and bacon come from, or what the main ingredient of yoghurt is. I know of a very middle-class child with professional parents who didn't recognise a potato, and I even met one mum who thought the dinky little bits of carrot in a single frozen vegetarian burger amounted to a portion of vegetables. And it's strange that we can be so squeamish about fresh raw meat and offal when we happily eat far more unsavoury bits of the animal (eyeballs, genitals, you name it) in burgers, kebabs and sausages.

The latest thing is for food to be colour coded with green spots for the healthier options and red for, presumably, foods which contain hydrogenated fats and unacceptably high levels of salt and sugar, but it goes without saying that if you stick to unprepared whole foods most of the time and give the ready meals a wide berth, colour coding is something you won't need to worry about.

When I was a child growing up in the 1970s, a healthy meal was meat and three veg followed by a fruit pudding; a takeaway meant the occasional trip to the fish and chip shop, and for something continental there was Batchelor's Savoury Rice and Vesta Curry. Now we can laugh, but people worried a lot less about food in those days; no one obsessed about their five portions a day, far more people stayed effortlessly slim, women apparently had smaller waistlines, obesity and obesity-related diseases were a lot less common, if not virtually unheard of, and a seriously overweight child was rarer than a white Christmas.

Much has been made in the past about the history of our unhealthy British diet, but it doesn't seem to me to have been too bad for what was, traditionally, a skinny population inhabiting a chilly little island off the North Sea. We may have had something to learn about the way we cooked our vegetables (like how to steam instead of boiling them to death), but what's wrong with potatoes, puddings and pies, as long as you're eating your greens? For my money, a proper home-cooked meal – with or without chips – is worth a dozen fast food hits that leave you with nothing but a craving for something sweet and a raging thirst.

Miracle foods come and go, but whether the current flavour of the month is wheat grass, alfalfa sprouts or Goji berries, the secret of feeding good food to your family without chaining yourself to the kitchen, depriving your children of the things they like to eat and driving yourself round the bend is that really, there *is* no secret. The answer was here all along.

THE STUMBLING BLOCKS... WHAT PUTS YOU OFF?

Whenever I come across a recipe containing mace (a spice made from the husk of a nutmeg apparently), a liqueur, or some other exotic, hard-to-get-hold-of ingredient I know I'll never use again, I immediately lose interest. One of my friends said she's put off by arty photographs of vegetables tied up in little parcels and anything else that looks too fiddly and refined, and to those two objections I would add recipes with too many ingredients, or too many stages from start to finish; something with a long preparation *and* a long cooking time (one or the other is just about okay), anything that requires a piece of equipment I don't have and probably haven't heard of, and, not having a dishwasher, anything that uses lots of pots and pans and makes too much washing up. I've also got an irrational fear of recipes containing gelatine for some reason, a perfectly rational fear of soufflés, and until quite recently I'd steer well clear of lentils if they had to be soaked overnight. Why, I don't know, since putting lentils in a bowl of cold water and rinsing them in a sieve takes about the same amount of time and energy as making a cup of tea, and I do that all the time.

It's all very well for celebrity chefs to say they want to get women back into the kitchen; what they don't seem to realise is that many people, myself included, owning nothing more sophisticated than a four-sided cheese grater, feel ruthlessly excluded by references to blini pans, griddles and pasta-making machines before we even start. Having said that, if you're serious about improving your family's eating habits, there are a few pieces of equipment you can't afford to be without, and in homes that have wide-screen TV, DVDs, iPods and game consoles in every room, none of them is exactly hi-tech.

An electric hand whisk is perfect for making cakes, among other things, while a food processor or blender (preferably 2 litre plus) is good for mixing, beating and liquidizing large quantities of anything and everything. The price of electrical goods is always coming down, so you shouldn't have any trouble finding these things for sale at around £5 for a hand whisk and £20 for a food processor. On the manual side, all the mixing bowls, casserole dishes, saucepans, cake tins, whisks, spoons and any other bits and pieces you need can be bought dirt cheap from the local supermarket or pound shop.

If you already have the right equipment and it's lack of confidence more than anything that keeps you from being more adventurous in the kitchen, all I can say is, there's nothing to worry about. It's practically unheard of for anyone to poison their family (by accident anyway) and you're unlikely to experience anything worse than a burnt saucepan, or food that's a bit browner around the edges than it was meant to be. Learning to cook is a bit like learning to drive; it only looks difficult from the outside. Once you realise you're the one in control of the machinery and not the other way round, there's nothing to it.

Don't worry about spending too many lonely hours in the kitchen on your own either. For one thing, there's nothing to stop you listening to the radio or having the television on if you need company; you can also drink alcohol and use your mobile while operating a food processor without breaking the law. It's even better if you can get the kids to help, which doesn't mean you have to let them waste your valuable time and make a mess of the kitchen while you grit your teeth and smile indulgently like an imaginary, perfect mother in a TV commercial. What you need is an assistant; someone to get the stuff out of the fridge for you, fetch whatever you need, open the packets, put the vegetable peelings in the right bin, (careful now) help with the tidying up and stir whatever you're cooking while you save all the best jobs for yourself. Not only is it possible to cut the preparation time right down, the children are picking up a set of good practical skills in the process, without even realising you're teaching them a lesson. How perfect is that?

But no matter how good your intentions are, there are bound to be times when it all goes pear-shaped and you find yourself eating cream crackers and cheese for dinner three nights in a row, usually when you're going through that stage of ferrying the children from one place to another after school and the family can't all be in the same place until bedtime (yours, usually). But there's always a solution to the eternal time problem, regardless of whether you're a full-time housewife or a working mum, it's just a case of finding out what works best for you. My advice is to cook more and do less ironing (or none at all) and think about what to eat in advance when you *do* have a bit of time. And if you really are that high-powered at work you must be paying someone else to look after your children part of the time, in which case, surely you established that they know what to do with the healthy food in your kitchen before you hired them?

Some people say we've lost a whole generation, if not two, to the fast food culture and there's little hope of things changing for the better in future, but I'm more optimistic than that. For one thing, the social and economic advantages of cooking and eating in your own home speak for themselves. Not 20 years ago, people were predicting we'd be getting all our reading material from the internet by now and that books would be obsolete, but there's no sign of that happening any time soon. With one health scare after another (BSE, foot-and-mouth, GM foods...) and so much evidence pointing to the ill-effects a terrible diet is having on our children, it can only be a matter of minutes before the tide turns back in favour of home cooking once and for all. Who knows? In five years' time, fast food outlets could be disappearing at the same rapid rate they were once springing up on the site of every derelict pub and petrol station in Britain.

What worries me more than anything about the current can't cook won't cook situation is that future generations of boys are going to grow up and not be able to irritate their wives by reminiscing about Yorkshire pudding and apple pie the way their mums used to make it. What will they say instead? *'Can you put this in the microwave like she did?'* It just doesn't have the same ring to it somehow, and that's a shame for all of us.

A WORD ABOUT WEIGHT LOSS

This is a recipe book, not a diet book, but there's no getting away from it; if you switch from commercially prepared and processed food to mostly healthy ingredients, and stop fretting about what you can and can't eat, you and your family are bound to lose weight, look better, feel fitter, have more energy – and be happier. Apart from eating poor quality food, nothing is more likely to make you put on weight than constant, miserable, half-hearted attempts to stop eating the things you like.

I don't think it's worth torturing yourself trying to resist the occasional craving for something 'unhealthy', whether it's fast food, drinks or sweets. But realistically, genuine cravings don't happen every day unless you're pregnant, and nobody puts on weight by eating a few chocolate bars, or a takeaway once a week. To pile on the pounds, you have to be eating chronically badly practically all the time.

When you stop and think about how you feel two hours after a fast food meal (hungry, thirsty and desperate for something sweet) compared with how you feel when you've eaten something truly nourishing, the advantages of real food over junk should be obvious. I don't know why we expect to have to suffer to be healthy when the opposite is true. It stands to reason that food that makes you *feel* good – in the long term, not just while you're eating it – must also be good *for* you. And whatever makes you *feel* lousy...

It's hardly rocket science, is it?

p.s. fizzy drinks...

On the subject of bad eating habits, it's impossible to ignore what must be the most pointless and easily avoidable evil of them all. Fizzy drinks.

Forget chocolate, chips and bacon sandwiches; even a burger with snotty, bright orange cheese and rubbery bits of gherkin has a certain appeal at times. But what's with the carbonated water? I don't get it. Fizzy drinks are either pretty bland or sickly sweet; too gassy, full of sugar or artificial sweeteners, and not only do they *not* do what they're supposed to, they actually make you thirstier than you were to start with, so you have to drink even more. It's brilliant! For the manufacturers, it's brilliant. Not so great for you, your weight, your teeth and your general health. Yet countless thousands or, God forbid, millions of people still drink this stuff every single day. And from what I've seen and heard, some people hardly drink anything else. Why?

EVERYDAY ESSENTIALS

The same ingredients crop up time and time again in these recipes. Keeping a few basic essentials in the cupboard means never having to say you're sorry but it's cornflakes for dinner again tonight...

Non-perishables

All the items listed below have a long shelf life, and as well as having a huge number of uses most of them are also *very* cheap, so you'll always have something to make a meal out of.

TINS: sardines, tuna, corned beef, chopped tomatoes, sweetcorn, vegetables, fruit, beans, beans, beans and more beans.

DRIED FRUIT: apricots, prunes, raisins and cranberries... N.B. *Dried bananas, apple and pineapple tend to be loaded with sugar, so unless you really struggle to get your children to eat fruit any other way, you're better off with fresh, or even tinned.*

RICE: white long grain and brown wholegrain. Pasta. Couscous.

FLOUR: plain, self-raising, wholemeal.

SUGAR: soft brown sugar, white sugar (granulated or caster).

OIL: any vegetable, corn or sunflower oil, plus olive oil and sesame oil.

Lemon juice, lime juice, vinegar (malt and cider).

Tubes of tomato puree, garlic puree and mustard.

STOCK CUBES: beef, pork, lamb, chicken and vegetable. N.B. *The cheapest ones contain too much salt, and as stock cubes don't cost much to begin with you may as well buy better ones. Knorr stock cubes are my favourite, and if they're good enough for Marco Pierre White...* Also instant gravy granules, Marmite, Bovril or Vegemite, and soy sauce.

Herbs & Spices

What on earth did we all do before the use of herbs and spices in everyday cooking finally caught on with the great British public? I remember when spice racks first started popping up in domestic kitchens in the 1970s, like the latest fashion accessory. Until then, the average family had never experienced anything more exotic than mint (with roast lamb) or mixed spice and cinnamon in homemade fruit cake. Now, most people have herbs and spices at home – but some people still aren't using them.

Herbs and spices add tremendous depth and flavour to all kinds of sweet and savoury foods, and nobody – whether you're wildly enthusiastic about cooking, or a bit on the lazy side like me – should be without them. (Every supermarket has a huge selection right next to the Oxo cubes, so you can't miss them.)

Tomato ketchup has its uses, but smother your dinner in tomato ketchup and all it tastes of is tomato ketchup, whereas herbs and spices complement and enhance the flavour of the food itself, without necessarily making it too strong and spicy. Don't worry about a rebellion at home if you haven't used them much before. Once your family gets used to eating food that actually tastes of something, they won't feel the need for a sugar and salt laden chemical fast food hit anywhere near as often as they would if they were still eating a lot of processed junk.

Fresh herbs can also be bought in the supermarket, although the range tends to be more limited, but if you want to use fresh instead of dried herbs in any of these recipes, that's even better. (I swear one day I'm going to buy only fresh herbs from a roadside market in a remote village somewhere in France – or grow my own. But for me, for now, without a pestle and mortar to my name, it's mostly dried herbs and ground spices out of a box, I'm afraid.)

Advice about which herbs and spices go well with certain foods is nearly always printed on the packaging you buy them in, but for the record, here are a few of the most popular and versatile ones, and a rough idea of how you can use them.

GINGER: Warm and spicy, especially good with lemon, lime juice, or brown sugar in stir fries, curries, cakes, biscuits, drinks and soup – you name it.

CURRY POWDER/CHILLI POWDER: Usually sold in mild, medium and hot. I tend to buy hot because, rightly or wrongly, I can't help feeling I must be getting more spice for my money that way. If I want a milder flavour I just use a bit less...

CUMIN: Boosts the flavour of curry and chilli powder and adds something extra.

CORIANDER: Great in curries, Mexican dishes, carrot and other orange vegetable soups.

PARSLEY: Sprinkled over tomato, potato, egg, cheese and fish dishes.

CHIVES: Omelettes, potato salad, vegetables dishes.

ROSEMARY: Roast lamb, Shepherd's Pie, some chicken dishes; good with roast potatoes.

SAGE: Great with pork, sausages and onions; homemade stuffing.

TARRAGON: Some fish and most chicken dishes (also good mixed with the breadcrumb coating on chicken goujons).

PAPRIKA: Subtly different from CAYENNE PEPPER (which is more fiery where paprika is milder and sweeter), to us amateurs the two are practically interchangeable, so I use paprika more often, in casseroles and goulash and on potato wedges.

MIXED HERBS: A good all-round substitute when you've run out of everything else.

MIXED SPICE: Good in cakes and biscuits, and as an alternative to ALL SPICE – which is similar but sharper; tasting more heavily of cloves – in some savoury dishes; stir fries, for example.

CINNAMON: Sweet and spicy, perfect with apples in cakes, puddings and biscuits.

NUTMEG: Good with spinach – especially where spinach is one of the main ingredients – and perfect in spicy fruit cakes, biscuits and banana smoothies.

One more thing I couldn't live without...

Natural bio live yoghurt has 101 uses in curries, soups, sauces, cakes and smoothies, as well being perfect with fruit, nuts and honey or on its own for breakfast, dessert, or a quick snack. I've never found anything better than Yeo Valley bio live yoghurts (natural and fruit). One helping is all you need to get the right balance of probiotics, without wasting money on fashionable, fruit-flavoured 'healthy' yoghurt drinks.

Salt

I never cook vegetables in salted water because I don't think it makes any difference to the flavour, especially if you add a little salt to your meal at the table, which is why a lot of these recipes don't include salt where you might expect to find it – in some of the sauces and most of the cakes, pastry and batter mixtures, for example. However, if you want to add a pinch of salt when you're cooking vegetables, fine, but don't overdo it with potatoes; they absorb a lot of salt from the water, which you're probably better off without.

Alcohol

Some of the recipes in this book contain a certain amount of alcohol. I never worried about letting my children eat food cooked with wine, sherry, cider or brandy, even when they were very young, but it's a personal decision, so put the alcohol in or leave it out; whatever you think is appropriate. If you don't buy much alcohol but like the idea of adding a splash of something to certain recipes, I think sherry has more uses than anything else, in everything from soup to puddings – or you could buy spirits in miniature bottles.

NOTES ON PREPARING VEGETABLES

I didn't have a clue about fennel before Jamie Oliver came along, and when I finally stumbled across it in the supermarket I wasn't sure what to do with it, so just in case, here's everything you to wanted to know about preparing and cooking vegetables but were afraid to ask.

ARTICHOKES: Remove the stalk and the tough or damaged outer leaves, then wash well, slice into quarters lengthways and get rid of the hairy centre bit, or 'choke". *To cook:* In fact, there are no recipes containing artichokes in this book, but if that wasn't enough to put you off and you feel like adding artichokes to soup, stews or casseroles, good luck to you.

ASPARAGUS: Cut off the hard ends to make all the asparagus spears the same length (although the supermarket should have already done this) and wash in cold water. (Only in season from middle of May to June.) *To cook:* Simmer gently in boiling water for 5–10 minutes, or place in a casserole dish with a lid, cover with a little cold water and cook in the microwave for 3 –4 minutes.

AUBERGINE: Top and tail; cut into thin slices and soak in a bowl of salty water for about 10 minutes, then strain away the brown, salty water and dry with kitchen paper, or an old, clean tea towel. *To cook:* Deep-fry the slices in very hot oil – about 3 inches (6 cm) deep will do; you don't need to fill the whole pan – as quickly as you can to stop them soaking up too much oil.

BEETROOT: Remove the long root and a bit of the stalk, wash and cut into quarters, but don't bother to peel. *To cook:* Bring to the boil in cold water and simmer gently for a good half an hour, then the skin can easily be rubbed off. Can be eaten at this stage, or drizzled with olive oil and roasted in the oven.

BUTTERNUT SQUASH: Wash and cut about 1 inch (1.5 cm) off either end. Cut in half lengthways; scrape out the foamy inner bit and remove the pips. Peel each half with a potato peeler or sharp knife (the skin is very tough), then cut into chunks. Alternatively, cut into chunks and cook the squash *first*, removing the skin after cooking when the squash is much softer. *To cook:* Boil and mash with butter and milk (starting in cold water, as with boiled potatoes) or drizzle with olive oil and roast in the oven.

CARROTS: No need to peel carrots; just top and tail, give them a quick scrape with a sharp vegetable knife and rinse in cold water. *To cook:* Start with cold water, bring to the boil and simmer gently for a few minutes until carrots are *barely* soft, with a bit of crunch left.

CELERIAC: Wash, peel and cut into chunks, or grate to have raw in salads (mixed with a little lemon juice to prevent discolouration).
To cook: Bring to the boil and simmer for 15–20 minutes until tender.

COURGETTES: Wash, top and tail. Depending on the size of the vegetable, cut into rounds, or cut lengthways once or twice, then slice from one end to the other to make it into halves or quarters. *To cook:* Warm oil or butter; add straight to the pan in stir fries and sauces (at same stage as onions and/or peppers) and cook for 10–15 minutes until soft.

FENNEL: Wash, trim and slice lengthways, or chop like an onion. The feathery bit at the top can also be chopped up and used in salads and sauces. *To cook:* Fry in butter or oil for a few minutes until soft.

PUMPKIN: *(see butternut squash above)*. *To cook:* Roast, boil and mash, or grate raw pumpkin to make pumpkin muffins.

A note on quantities and sizes used in this book

Unless otherwise specified, the quantities of vegetables and seasoning, etc in each recipe are purely a matter for the reader to decide upon, depending on the size and age of your family, appetites, and so on...

Most recipes state how many people it will serve, but sometimes, this has not been included, as again it depends on your particular family, whether you are serving the recipe as a main course or accompaniment, or simply how large a portion of cake, pudding, etc you want!

One final note, some recipes use a 'standard' tin, this means a 14 oz (410 g) sized tin.

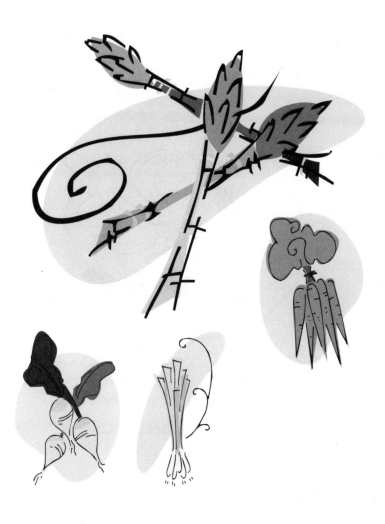

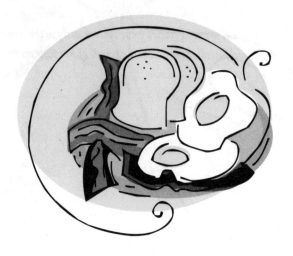

"All happiness depends
on a leisurely breakfast."

John Gunther

Wake up to breakfast

Breakfast wasn't very exciting when I was a child; toast and cereal just about had it covered in our house, so once I started going to work early in the morning I dispensed with breakfast altogether and ate a couple of Kit Kats on the bus. Then I left home and breakfast became a cup of tea and a cigarette, followed by another cup of tea and a cigarette at the office. In fact, I didn't really take breakfast seriously until I was pregnant for the first time in my twenties – and then it was a struggle to keep down one Weetabix.

Lots of people, especially children, dread eating first thing in the morning, but endless research has shown how important breakfast is. Having witnessed the effects of going without food on tired, listless and irritable kids, I agree that getting them to eat something before they leave the house makes a huge difference, not only to their happiness and well-being, but to the way they behave and perform at school, so it's worth getting into good habits as soon as you can.

There's nothing wrong with toast and cereal of course, but there are plenty of alternatives, so try and make breakfast a bit more interesting and less of a chore by ringing the changes and finding out what your children like, what they don't like, and what they wouldn't eat if it was the only thing between them and total starvation.

If you want them to eat something they haven't tried before and you're not sure how they're going to react, give them the chance to try it first at the weekend or in the holidays, rather than on a school morning when you're pushed for time and already have a hundred-and-one things to worry about.

EVERYDAY BREAKFASTS

Cereal

I think it's fair to say you can separate cereal into two camps; the goodies, made entirely from whole grains with little, or no, added salt and sugar, and the baddies, which contain a lot of extra sugar, and in some cases as much salt as you'd find in a bag of crisps.

I suppose any cereal has to be better than nothing because they all contain added vitamins and are eaten with milk (and if you get into the good habit of not giving children extra sugar from the very beginning, they'll never miss it). There's nothing to stop you reading the labels on every box in the supermarket if you feel like it but, as a general rule, the less fancy looking the cereal, the healthier it's going to be. Anything frosted, flavoured, coloured, coated in honey or mixed with chocolate chips and other bits and pieces is certain to contain some or all of the things you want to avoid, so here's a quick guide to your best bets.

PORRIDGE: All porridge, any porridge; from a box, from a bag, or an individual sachet. There shouldn't be any added sugar in porridge oat cereals, even the one aimed specifically at children, and now porridge can be made in the microwave you don't even have the bother of cleaning the saucepan afterwards.

KELLOGG'S ALL BRAN: Greatly improved since the days when it tasted exactly like minced cardboard, but if you still can't bear to eat it on its own (I can't), make a delicious fruit and bran loaf with it instead *(see Wholesome Cakes in Chapter 8: Let Them Eat Cake)*.

SHREDDED WHEAT: The bite-size version is especially good for kids, and this is one cereal that doesn't go soggy in the milk.

MUESLI: With or without added sugar, there are so many healthy ingredients in muesli, does it really matter?

WEETABIX: Make it more interesting for children by pouring on a fruit smoothie, or milk flavoured with a spoonful of Nesquik, rather than plain milk. (Take the Weetabix Challenge — you must have seen the TV adverts.)

Fruit

If you haven't eaten fruit for breakfast before because you're worried you'll be starving long before lunch, give it a try; I bet you find a good helping of fruit (especially with yoghurt) fills you up far more effectively than a bowl of soggy cereal.

In fact, fruit is a really easy option at breakfast time, especially in the spring and summer months, and I've found that even children who don't normally go a bundle on fruit often find a few slices of banana with a small spoonful of yoghurt and honey less daunting than a piece of toast or a bowl of cereal. Not only does it look more inviting, it's nice to have something sweet when you've got a dry, early morning taste in your mouth. (If you're worried about brushing your teeth too soon after having fruit, eat a small piece of cheese to neutralise the acid in your mouth and protect the enamel, then wait a couple of minutes. The same rule applies any time you've eaten food containing a lot of acid; I always gave my children a piece of cheese after a marathon sweet-eating session — of which there were many — and it seems to have worked for them so far.)

Just a few slices or chunks of fruit, or a combination of fruits, e.g. banana, apple, pear, melon, kiwi fruit, grapes or berries, with live yoghurt (natural or fruit) and a teaspoonful of honey drizzled over the top.

Half a grapefruit or an orange cut into segments and sprinkled with a very little sugar. Flash the fruit under the grill to melt the sugar and take the chill off if you like, especially in the winter when cold fruit isn't so appealing. (If you buy the sweeter varieties of grapefruit you shouldn't even need to add sugar.)

Tinned prunes. Soft, sweet and easy to eat. Most tinned prunes I've come across aren't even particularly wrinkled, despite what their bad reputation suggests. (Eat five, then if you do 'Tinker, Tailor' with the stones, it always come out 'rich man'.)

Fruit smoothies. The possibilities are endless *(see Chapter 7: Can't Cook? Don't Cook!)*.

Cake

Cake is the answer to a parent's prayers on those cold, dark winter mornings when it's an effort getting out of bed on time, no one fancies fruit, and you don't want to make anything more complicated than a cup of tea. When you think about it, plenty of Europeans with far fewer health problems than we have in this country eat cakes, croissants and jam for breakfast all the time, and I don't see a problem as long as children have a small glass of milk or fresh juice with it.

Bran loaf, rock buns, fruit and muesli muffins, bread pudding, flapjacks, apple, ginger, carrot or plum cake *(see Wholesome Cakes in Chapter 8: Let Them Eat Cake)* or cheese and courgette scones *(see Cooking with Children in Chapter 8: Let Them Eat Cake)* all do the trick.

Eggs

Eggs are so versatile, and in their simplest forms they only take a very few minutes to cook.

BOILED: Everyone has a theory on the best way to boil an egg, and now there's more than one gadget on the market to do the job for you. Assuming you're not spoilt and selfish enough to have your butler produce six boiled eggs in a row for you to choose from, all you have to do is start with cold water, a teaspoon of salt and a drop of vinegar in the smallest saucepan you've got; then bring to the boil and simmer gently for 2 ½ minutes for a very soft boiled egg, i.e. white just firm and yolk very runny. If you're doing several eggs at once and everyone likes their egg a different way, follow the same procedure and remove all the eggs from the water at the same time. Eggs carry on cooking in their shells, so take the tops off the 'soft' eggs straight away; anyone who wants a harder egg can wait another two minutes while they eat a piece of toast, before taking the top off their egg.

POACHED EGGS: I've tried poaching eggs in the microwave as well as in a pan specially designed for the job, but I still think the easiest way by far is just to break the egg into a cup and drop it straight into a saucepan of lightly salted, gently boiling water; about 2 minutes for a firm white and soft yolk, 3 – 4 minutes for a firm yolk.

OPEN HOUSE EGGS: Warm enough oil to just cover the bottom of a frying pan; cut a hole in a piece of bread with a cup or glass and put both pieces of bread into the pan. Break an egg into a cup and drop it into the hole in the slice of bread. After a couple of minutes, flip everything over and fry for another couple of minutes. Squeeze tomato sauce onto the egg, replace the circle and serve.

SCRAMBLED EGGS: Add a good splash of milk to make the eggs go further (for me, scrambled eggs without milk are too rich anyway) and for speed, scramble them in a large, non-stick, shallow frying pan – as opposed to a regular, deep-sided saucepan – with a tablespoonful of melted butter.

Kippers

Boil-in-the-bag kippers take about 10 minutes; sprinkle them with lemon juice (and dried parsley) and eat with brown bread and butter.

Avocado Sandwiches

Mash an avocado (or two, according to how many sandwiches you want to make), spread on brown bread and butter and cut the crusts off. Avocados are the perfect good mood food; nice and easy for little mouths to swallow first thing in the morning.

Pancakes

If you can't bring yourself to make batter and get a pan dirty before breakfast on a school morning, make a stack of pancakes in advance and freeze them.

TO MAKE ABOUT A PINT OF BATTER (6 – 12 PANCAKES, DEPENDING ON THICKNESS OF PANCAKES AND SIZE OF PAN):
4–5 very heaped tablespoons of plain flour
2 eggs
½ pint (250 ml) milk

METHOD
1. Sift the flour into a bowl or a large mixing jug (2 pint plus),make a well in the centre, add the eggs and about half the milk, start whisking with a small hand whisk or fork and gradually add the rest of the milk. Thin with a little more milk if necessary. Transfer the batter into a jug, which will make it easier to pour into the frying pan.
2. The secret of perfect pancakes is a very hot pan and no surplus oil sloshing around, so warm enough oil to cover the bottom of the frying pan, then pour the oil into a clean cup to be used again, and give the pan a quick wipe over with kitchen roll.
3. Pour in enough batter to make a pancake, tipping the pan as you go to get the bottom of the pan covered as quickly as possible.

4. As soon as the surface of the pancake is completely dry, run a knife around the edge and turn it over, or toss it by holding the pan away from you, shaking the pancake towards the far end as far as it will go without falling out, and flipping it over in one deft movement. (N.B. Pour a little more oil from the cup into the pan after every couple of pancakes, heat thoroughly, then wipe the pan almost dry with kitchen roll.)

TO FREEZE:

1. Make the pancakes as described above, layer them with clingfilm when they've cooled (which only takes a few minutes), then put the whole lot in a large food bag and freeze.
2. No need to defrost them; place each pancake on a plate – or two pancakes on one plate, a little apart – and microwave on high for 1 – 2 minutes.

PEANUT BUTTER PANCAKES:

I thought of making pancakes with peanut butter as a way of adding protein, otherwise pancakes can be a bit lightweight when you've got a busy day ahead and no way of knowing when you'll be able to eat again.

I use smooth peanut butter – it blends easily with the batter in seconds – but I don't see why you couldn't use crunchy peanut butter instead if you prefer it.

1. Make batter in the usual way, with a bit less milk, and use a fork to whisk a dessert spoonful of peanut butter into the mixture at the end – roughly 1 dessert spoon for ½ pint (250 ml) of batter. (Add more milk if the batter needs thinning.)
2. Make pancakes in the usual way and serve with slices of banana and maple or golden syrup.

WEEKEND BREAKFASTS

Unless you're super-efficient and get up at the crack of dawn, some breakfasts are better left until the weekend.

Eggs Florentine

Make cheese sauce in the usual way; mixing a heaped tablespoon of flour with about 1oz (25g) of melted butter in a saucepan, cooking for a minute, then adding approximately ½ pint (250 ml) of milk, a handful of grated cheese and whisking continually until the sauce thickens. Keep the sauce warm and cover with clingfilm or a couple of tablespoons of milk to prevent a skin forming while you wash and cook the spinach, preferably in the microwave in a casserole dish with a lid, and poach the eggs in boiling water. Serve the eggs on a bed of spinach with the cheese sauce poured over the top.

Hash Browns, Bacon & Beans

As an alternative to grilling or frying, place bacon on a lightly greased tray at the top of the oven and cook on Gas Mark 6 (200°C) for about 20 minutes – no need to turn it over. If you're making hash browns, fry them lightly on both sides and finish them off in the middle of the oven, warming the baked beans up in a casserole dish with a lid on at the bottom. Needless to say, homemade hash browns are infinitely superior to their supermarket equivalent (*see Chapter 9: Not Only But Also*).

The Healthiest 'Fry-up' Possible (with the least amount of washing up)

1. Cook sausages in the oven in a very large ovenproof dish (preferably Pyrex, it's easier to clean), adding the bacon about

halfway through the sausages' cooking time.

2. Put baked beans and tinned plum tomatoes in a casserole dish with a lid on at the bottom of the oven 10 minutes after you put the bacon in.

3. Half-fill a large saucepan with boiling water from the kettle and put it on a low heat while you make toast.

4. Poach the eggs in the boiling water for a very few minutes, by which time everything should be ready – and that's it!

ALSO TRY...

Baked Apples (*see Chapter 6: Join the Pudding Club*), Kedgeree and Cheese & Onion Tomatoes (*see Chapter 3: Make Dinner, Not Excuses*).

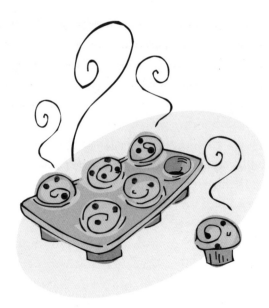

"Ask your child what he wants for
dinner only if he's buying."

Fran Lebowitz

Little gems and tough cookies

Feeding your children good food is every parent's obligation. In fact, we all come from a long line of parents who fed their children, so why now, when we're swamped with so much advice and information about our food and the number of fat grams and calories it contains, does hardly a week go by without another deeply depressing story about morbidly obese children whose parents can't, or won't, stop feeding them a non-stop diet of processed rubbish?

Apparently, British teenagers are the first generation to be less healthy than their parents, and I read recently that increasing numbers of children are becoming anorexic, some of them, unbelievably, as young as six- and seven- years-old.

But maybe it's not surprising that kids are resorting to starving themselves when so many adults are permanently stressed out and pre-occupied with food. If the parents are anxious and confused – withholding treats with one hand and feeding their children processed rubbish with the other – while their teachers search their lunchboxes for illicit chocolate biscuits and packets of crisps, what are they supposed to think?

Constantly subjected to images of size zero models and the idealistic, unrealistic zeal of humourless healthy eating gurus on one hand; continually bombarded by the message that junk food and fizzy drinks are cool on the other – is it any wonder that going without nourishment altogether is starting to seem like the only alternative to obesity in the minds of impressionable young children?

But despite this grim picture, we can count ourselves lucky that you don't need to be an expert on *anything* to feed your children a healthy, balanced diet with very little money and hardly any time, even if you have a tiny kitchen, only three saucepans (one with an ill-fitting lid) and no fancy gadgets unless you count the garlic crusher. Although it sometimes feels like an uphill struggle, whether your children are little gems who eat whatever you put in front of them, tough cookies who seem to leave more on the plate than you put there or, like most kids, a combination of the two, cooking real food is nowhere near as exhausting, tricky or unrewarding as some people make it out to be.

Finally, and speaking from experience, it doesn't matter where or how you live, feeding your children good food and laying the groundwork for the healthiest possible future is something that every one of us has in our power to get right.

FUSSY EATERS

There can't be many children who *don't* go through a fussy stage, whether it's one type of food they don't like, food generally (heaven help you), or a particular time of day when they don't seem to want to eat anything.

Whatever it is, it's not worth losing your temper over; all that does is frighten the child and make the situation worse. Be prepared to be patient, even if you're feeling anxious, and remind yourself that the important thing is to encourage your children to eat, and eventually enjoy food, without turning mealtimes into a battleground, because if that happens, you really will have trouble on your hands.

I've found there are two schools of thought when it comes to persuading kids to eat. Either talk to them about their food; let them know exactly what it is and where it comes from, or try and disguise whatever they don't like so they end up eating some of the right foods without realising. It's a case of working out which way works best in your house, and at the risk of confusing the issue, you'll probably find it will be a little bit of both.

Just remember that children have seldom, if ever, starved themselves completely, or incurred any lasting damage to their health by refusing certain foods, even kids who exist on a diet of baked beans and jelly babies, or some other weird combination, for months at a time.

Of course it's better all round if they learn to like a wide variety of foods early on and, from a personal point of view, I don't see any harm in offering a reward in the form of a pudding, or a very few sweets after dinner every day if that helps. Having said that, it's a good idea to give fruit as a treat sometimes (especially in the summer months when the really good stuff is in season: strawberries, raspberries, cherries, peaches and plums, among other things) rather than the more obvious sweet treats, so children don't differentiate between nutritious and 'naughty but nice' things too soon, in which case they're naturally going to want the latter every time.

Like everything else in life it's a question of finding the right balance, so be firm without being too forceful and you'll soon be able to spot the difference between a child who genuinely dislikes something, and one who's just pushing his luck because he'd rather eat a bag of crisps than a bowl of soup.

There's no better way for children to develop good eating habits than watching their parents eat and enjoy food, so eat together as a family whenever you can, or if the children are very young and have dinner earlier than you, at least stay in the same room, and preferably sit down with them, so you can have a conversation and help them along if they're struggling.

Try not to fly off the handle when they refuse to eat something the first fifty-five times, and shower them with praise and admiration when they do try. It's easy to forget that children actually want to please their parents most of the time (children under the age of twelve anyway), so make them feel good about themselves and lay off the guilt. There'll be plenty of time for that later on when they're selfish, ungrateful teenagers who treat the house like a hotel and don't appreciate anything you've done for them.

Tips

Impose strict limits on juice and squash and banish fizzy drinks altogether, except for parties and special occasions. I've lost count of the number of very young children I've seen guzzling vast quantities of drink, and then, to the surprise and despair of their parents, not being able to eat anything. Avoid giving small children anything to drink except water and a certain amount of milk for as long as possible, and if you must give them juice, dilute it with as much water as you can get away with. Even expensive, unsweetened fruit juice can damage their teeth and too much liquid sloshing around in their stomachs takes the edge off their appetite. Never serve soft drinks at mealtimes either, just a jug of water, with or without ice. If children are genuinely thirsty they *will* drink water, or very diluted fruit juice, no two ways about it. This is one area where it pays to be really ruthless. It's up to you to put your foot down.

Keep portions small. It's better to give a child a tiny amount so they can ask for more than put them off with too much food at the start.

Whenever you want them to eat food they say they don't like, or just something new that they haven't tried before, make sure you also give them something you know they do like. (Tempt them with chips and they might just eat the other vegetables on their plate without complaining.)

Try not to separate food into 'good' and 'bad' or 'adult' and 'kiddie' food and, no matter what their age, eat at least some of the same foods as your children at every meal.

If it's the texture of certain foods more than the taste that's putting your child off, make fruit and vegetable smoothies in a blender for them to drink through a straw.

Keep trying new things and don't be afraid to re-introduce food they didn't like the first time round. Getting your kids into good eating habits is like teaching them road safety. You don't bring the subject up once or twice at the beginning and assume they've learnt it; you still say 'mind the road' every time they go near it – even when they're old enough to drive on it.

Some sweet treats are less harmful than others, so give children small amounts of chocolate rather than hard, sugar-coated candy whenever possible. Ice pops and plain lollies are another good bet for a relatively harmless sweet treat. In fact, it's a good idea to keep ice pops in the freezer all year round for when your kids are very sick or down with the flu. Slowly sucking an ice pop helps keep them hydrated when they can't eat or they're constantly throwing up.

For a savoury snack give them dry cereal or a few cheesy biscuits, instead of crisps.

Never, ever give a young child a whole packet of sweets or crisps in any case; split one packet between at least three kids and give each of them a tiny amount in a small bowl. If you've only got one child and you're trying not to fall into the trap of eating all their leftovers, seal the packet with sticky tape immediately, then put it back in the cupboard – and always buy the smallest packets in the first place.

Use a favourite doll or teddy as a prop. Whether you're potty-training, trying to get kids to take their medicine or encouraging them to eat, there's nothing most very young children like more than a game involving a loved and trusted toy.

Grow your own herbs or mustard and cress in a pot on the windowsill and cook as an activity (*see Cooking with Children in*

Chapter 8: Let Them Eat Cake) to get them interested in food and reduce the fear factor.

Have other kids over to eat with your children regularly so they can socialize and learn to associate food with happy occasions, instead of seeing every mealtime as an obstacle that has to be overcome as quickly as possible.

Separate the food on their plate into two piles and let your children choose to eat just one of them. Meet them halfway and none of you will be left feeling like the loser.

PACKED LUNCHES

Q: How do you make a reasonably nutritious packed lunch that won't reduce your child to tears of boredom or have you branded an unfit mother? It's no joke.

Once upon a time, all we had to worry about was the odd spilt drink or a squashed sandwich. Now, providing children with a packed lunch every day without finding the rotten remains hidden under the bed six weeks later or falling foul of the Lunchbox Police is more hazardous than a trip to Mars – and put one of those in their lunchbox at your peril.

Unless you're one of those lucky parents whose children's school prepares proper, decent food on the premises – or you couldn't care less – the chances are you'll find yourself making packed lunches at least some of the time for a good few years. And no, I don't think a Mars Bar is the answer either, but I don't buy the 'one size fits all' philosophy of schools who invent ridiculous rules about what you can and can't feed your children as a smokescreen for the unpalatable truth, which is; the food they provide is often even less healthy than crisps and chocolate and they can't be bothered to address the problem any other way. (One teacher I know of at a very PC primary school, which has

'Healthy Schools Status,' whatever that means, allows the children's lunchboxes to be kept right next to the radiator.)

I agree that if you can't be bothered to try and feed your children something healthy at least some of the time you deserve a kick up the backside, but most of us *do* care very much, and I don't think anyone is in a better position than the parents to predict what their children *will actually eat*. It's all very well advising people to pack fruit salad and sandwiches full of lettuce and tomato, but there's no getting away from it, fruit doesn't always taste so good in a plastic box, and salad sandwiches go soggy long before lunchtime, no matter what.

Children can be very conservative in their eating habits and it's frustrating if they insist on taking cream crackers and jam for lunch every day, but if they've had breakfast and you know they'll eat a proper meal later on, it's nobody else's business. Nor do I think it's necessarily a bad thing to pack a small bag of crisps or a chocolate biscuit in addition to the main course. I always gave my children crisps and biscuits on condition that they ate at least half the sandwich and a bit of fruit first, and if they didn't have time for the treat I always let them eat it later on. Of course you need a bit of trust for this to work, but as a veteran packed lunch maker of many years' standing, I believe it generally *does* work – and any dinner lady worth her salt will see to it that no child gets the wrapper off a chocolate biscuit while there's an untouched sandwich or an apple in their lunchbox.

I was a school dinner lady some years ago and I saw lots of packed lunches which had obviously been lovingly prepared by health-conscious parents, but which also included crisps, biscuits, cakes and other now strictly forbidden items. I also saw some truly *dire* lunches – a single slice of cold, soggy toast, for example – which wouldn't break any of the new rules, but hardly qualifies as wholesome either. The other important point about rules and forbidden food is that whatever isn't allowed automatically becomes more desirable. At this rate we'll have a black market in Penguins and Jaffa Cakes run by nine-year-olds behind the disused bike sheds before we know it.

Another thing I've noticed over the years is that the way kids of all ages eat at home can be very different from the way they act in front of their friends, and let's face it, most dinner halls aren't exactly conducive to eating in peace and comfort. Then there's the time factor, the lure of the playground and the smell of school dinners to put them off, not to mention peer pressure, as in: *'Eugh, what is THAT? You're not eating it are you?'* I remember a ten-year-old girl telling one of my children that his mum didn't love him because he had own-brand crisps in his lunchbox instead of Walkers. Honestly. Another time I couldn't understand why my teenage son flatly refused to take smoked salmon sandwiches to school, which he loves, until, in a moment of sudden clarity I realised that eating dainty smoked salmon sandwiches at the local comprehensive was more likely to get him duffed up than going around with a sign on his back saying 'punch me'.

Let's be clear about one thing. When your children are in primary school, you do at least have half a chance to get it right. After that, peer pressure (especially with boys) kicks in so hard you'll be lucky if they eat or drink *anything* that isn't fizzy, fried or covered in sugar. Then all you can do is hope for the best and make sure they still eat the right food at home, where you still have *some* influence...

Tips

If you have to make sandwiches in advance, wrap them in foil and store them in the fridge.

Cut the crusts off if you think it helps – two sandwiches without crusts for older kids – it makes them easier to wolf down in a hurry, and they get to eat more of the best bit of the sandwich that way.

Prepare sandwich fillings the night before, i.e. mash tuna, grate cheese, etc, then you're already halfway there in the morning.

Buy lots of plastic boxes with tight-fitting lids in a variety of shapes and sizes; they come in handy for so many things (*see below*).

The Food

Don't stick to the same old white sliced. Even if your kids have sandwiches every day you can make them more interesting by varying the bread, as well as the filling. Granary, rye, wholemeal, white grain, half-and-half, pumpernickel, crusty rolls, cheesy rolls, bagels, wraps and croissants all work well with any of the following: cheese and pickle, tinned tuna or salmon mixed with sweetcorn and mayonnaise, ham and cream cheese, beef and watercress, avocado and bacon, slices of cold meatloaf and mustard...

Reduce the likelihood of a soggy outcome (slightly) by putting salad between two layers of filling, away from the bread. Even so, it has to be said that some salad stuff lasts better than others. I've never had much success with tomato and lettuce, but diced cucumber and peppers can be mixed with tuna and mayonnaise; also watercress or mustard and cress, and sweetcorn.

Pack slices of tomato and cucumber or lettuce and spinach in boxes with tight-fitting lids to be added to sandwiches or rolls at lunchtime.

Avoid anything that will smell, spill, or go off too quickly, especially in the summer. Egg sandwiches are out, and cartons of yoghurt generally don't last the course – plus there's a good chance that the lid will be pierced by a sharp object, covering everything with the contents.

Compartmentalized lunchboxes can be good for keeping everything separate and therefore less liable to damage.

Try the old trick of packing a carton of juice straight from the freezer to keep everything else in the lunchbox cool in the summer. By lunchtime, the drink will still be half-frozen and mushy like a Slush Puppy.

Instead of sandwiches try:

- Cold chicken drumsticks or homemade chicken nuggets with coleslaw (*see Chapter 3: Make Dinner, Not Excuses*).
- Sausage rolls and potato salad (*see Chapter 3: Make Dinner, Not Excuses*).
- Hummus or guacamole with carrot sticks and tortilla chips (*see Chapter 9: Not Only But Also*).
- Cold pizza.
- Pasta mixed with tuna, diced cucumber and sweetcorn.
- Rice salad (*see Chapter 3: Make Dinner, Not Excuses*).
- For slightly older kids, fill a thermos flask with hot soup or pasta and tomato sauce. This is definitely too nerdy for most teenagers, and even if it does work you'll probably find yourself replacing the broken flask at least once a term, but it's always worth a try.

Buy the smallest bananas, fun-size apples and seedless grapes, which are much more appealing and less daunting to children (not to mention plenty of adults).

Apples and bananas can get boring when there's nothing very exciting in season, so provide sticks of carrot, celery, cucumber, red and green peppers instead.

Don't forget dried fruit; raisins, prunes, apricots, dates, figs and cranberries.

Bend the no crisps or biscuits rule with homemade cheesy biscuits and wholesome cakes (*see Chapter 8: Let Them Eat Cake*).

Make fruit jelly in tiny plastic pots with tight-fitting lids the night before; they'll be set by the morning. (Give kids plastic spoons and forks if you find the contents of your cutlery drawer gradually disappearing without trace.)

If your children are desperate for something sweet and there's no ban on chocolate at their primary school include a couple of squares of good dark chocolate in their lunchbox to finish off with.

p.s. The very clever mother of one six-year-old boy I knew when I was a dinner lady used to leave funny little messages in his lunchbox, encouraging him to eat his food and enjoy it. Plenty of mothers, myself included, can only marvel at such devotion and presence of mind (my children would never have been able to read my terrible handwriting anyway) but, hey, it's a good idea. Maybe it could work for you.

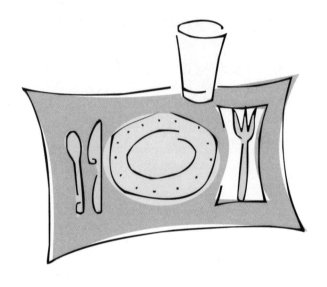

"But when the time comes that a man has had his dinner, then the true man comes to the surface."

Mark Twain

Make dinner, not excuses

MINCE

Mince may be the poor relation of beef, pork and lamb, but it certainly has its uses, not least because it's perfect for disguising large quantities of vegetables in. It's also very versatile and inexpensive and a good starting point for getting kids accustomed to the taste and smell of meat, assuming that's what you want to do.

Once again, as it's so affordable to begin with there's not much to be gained from buying the cheapest. However, regardless of what kind of mince you buy, you should always get rid of the extra fat by almost covering the pan with a lid once the meat is cooked, then tipping the pan and carefully straining off as much of the fatty liquid as you can. Liposuction for meat, in other words – and if you haven't done this before you'll be horrified at the amount of extra fat you could have been swallowing. *Eugh*.

Tips

Use a couple of tins of corned beef in Shepherd's Pie instead of minced lamb if you feel like something different.

Always dry-fry mince straight from the packet; even if the label says 'extra lean steak' it still contains more fat than you need.

Make leftover chilli or Bolognese go further by adding a couple of tins of chopped tomatoes and some more seasoning.

SHEPHERD'S PIE

Not long ago I read that when Jamie Oliver asked a young mum why she didn't make Shepherd's Pie for her kids she said it was 'too posh'.

Shepherd's Pie is a lot of things – delicious, cheap and easy to put together all year round – but posh? I don't think so.

There's no end to what you can add to the meat in Shepherd's Pie, so try finely chopped celery, a handful of frozen mixed vegetables, spinach, grated carrot, sweetcorn, or leftover vegetables (carrots, swede, cabbage or broccoli, for instance) cut into small pieces.

Instead of potato alone, use a mixture of potato and sweet potato or butternut squash for the topping; add an egg to make the potato drier and fluffier, or a spoonful of creamed cheese with parsley or chives, or just plain butter and milk.

Minced lamb is a bit more expensive than minced beef, (although not that much) so if you can't get lamb or you want to use minced beef instead, just add plenty of rosemary; hardly anyone will be able to tell the difference.

Serve with green vegetables, or just baked beans, and make extra gravy if you like a wet dinner.

SERVES 4–6:
1 lb (approx 450–500 g) minced lamb
1 onion, chopped
Mushrooms
Carrot, grated
Frozen sweetcorn
1 lamb, beef or vegetable stock cube (or a teaspoon of Marmite)
1 clove of garlic
Tomato puree
1 tbsp instant gravy granules
Dried rosemary

Potatoes: however many you think would make a serving of
   mash for each person
Splash of milk
Grated cheese, approx 1 oz (25 g)

METHOD
1. Peel potatoes, or wash them and leave them in their skins (*see
   page 102*), then cut them roughly into quarters and put them on
   the hob in a saucepan of fresh, cold water.
2. Dry-fry the meat in a very large pan on a low heat, breaking it
   up with a wooden spoon now and then, while you get the
   vegetables ready.
3. Add the onion and garlic to the pan as soon as you like, then add the
   mushrooms and grated carrot, stirring every now and then until the
   meat is almost cooked and you can clearly see the fatty juices.
4. Strain the fat off the meat (*see page 43*), then crumble in the
   stock cube and add the rosemary, a couple of handfuls of
   frozen sweetcorn and a tablespoonful of tomato puree.
5. Add a tablespoonful of instant gravy granules to thicken and
   then simmer for a few minutes until the potatoes are ready,
   then transfer the meat into a large ovenproof dish.
6. Drain and mash the potatoes with a lump of butter and a
   splash of milk; add the grated cheese, then spread the potato
   topping over the meat, and put in the oven on Gas Mark 5
   (190°C) for 15–20 minutes, or until the potatoes are brown
   and the gravy is bubbling.

MOUSSAKA

SERVES 6:
1 lb (450–500 g) minced lamb
1 onion, finely chopped

2 cloves of garlic
2 aubergines
4 medium-large potatoes
Mushrooms
1 lamb or beef stock cube
1 tsp all spice
Tomato puree
Very little water

FOR THE TOPPING:
1 pint (500 ml) warm milk
4 oz (100 g) butter
3 tbsp plain flour
2 egg yolks

METHOD
1. Cook the minced lamb in a very large saucepan with the finely chopped onion and garlic for a few minutes, then strain off the fatty liquid *(see page 43)*.
2. Crumble in the stock cube, add some tomato puree with the all spice and a very little water and stir well.
3. Meanwhile, peel and put the potatoes on to boil in a pan of fresh cold water; bring to the boil, simmer until soft, then allow to cool for a few minutes before cutting into thick slices.
4. Cut the aubergines into thinly sliced quarters and soak in a bowl of salty water for 5 minutes while you peel and finely slice the mushrooms.
5. Drain the aubergines thoroughly with a clean tea towel or kitchen roll, then deep fry in very hot oil and leave to drain on clean kitchen roll.
6. Put the fried aubergines in a bowl and mix with the sliced mushrooms. (The aubergines absorb so much oil there's no

need to fry the mushrooms as well.)
7. Layer the meat with the aubergines and mushrooms in a large ovenproof dish and finish with a layer of sliced potato.

TO MAKE THE TOPPING:
1 pint (500 ml) warm milk
4 oz (100 g) butter
3 tbsp plain flour
2 egg yolks

1. Melt the butter in a saucepan and warm the milk (in another saucepan, or in a large bowl in the microwave: approx 4 minutes on high).
2. Add the flour to the melted butter in the saucepan and stir over the heat for a minute, then pour in the warm milk, whisking all the time.
3. When the sauce starts to thicken, add the egg yolks and whisk for another minute.
4. Pour the topping over the moussaka and bake in the oven for 30 −40 minutes, Gas Mark 4 (180°C) until the sauce is bubbling and the topping has a golden crust.

CHILLI CON CARNE

As usual, the quantities here are all approximate, so add more, or less of the vegetables, according to what you have and what you like best; the same applies to the amount of chilli powder, cumin, etc. I always make more chilli then I need and keep (or freeze) some, which is why there's more meat here than in most other mince recipes; in fact, the quantities below should be enough to make two meals (accompanied by pasta, rice, salad and vegetables, etc) for a family of four.

2 lb (1 kg) lean minced beef
1 large onion
2 peppers, any colour
2 courgettes
Mushrooms
Spinach
1 tin of kidney beans
1 or 2 tins of plum or chopped tomatoes
Tomato puree
Garlic puree
Chilli powder
Pinch of curry powder
Cumin
1 beef stock cube
Basil

Method

1. Put the mince in a large, deep-sided pan on a low heat and let it brown slowly while you wash and chop the vegetables. (Break up the lumps of meat from time to time with a wooden spoon.)
2. When the meat is just about cooked, strain off the fatty liquid (*see page 43*) and add the peppers, courgettes, mushrooms, onion, herbs and spices and give it all a good stir.
3. Wash a generous handful of spinach and add to the meat with the tinned tomatoes; keep stirring and turn the heat right up to make it bubble. Thoroughly rinse the kidney beans in a sieve and put them in too.
4. Add enough tomato puree to thicken the sauce until it's the way you like it, then turn the heat right down, cover with a lid and simmer very gently for about half an hour.

HAMBURGERS

Use lean minced beef or buy the best steak you can afford and mince it in a blender or food processor at home. Add a finely chopped onion, a few herbs, and some breadcrumbs if you want to stretch the meat a bit further. You don't need a huge amount of meat to make a good hamburger, especially if you top it up with salad, real cheese (as opposed to processed slices, or that gunk from a plastic bottle...what exactly is that stuff, anyway?) and chunky homemade chips.

MAKES 6 GOOD-SIZED BURGERS:
2 lb (1 kg) minced beef or steak
1 large onion, finely chopped
1 egg to bind

OPTIONAL:
Paprika or cayenne pepper
Black pepper
Parsley
Breadcrumbs

METHOD
1. Squish everything together in a large bowl and pat the mixture into burger shapes with your hands, making them as large and thin as you can without them falling apart. (Only use flour if you feel you can't manage without; you don't really need it.)
2. For best results put the burgers under the grill on the highest setting and cook on both sides for a few minutes until they're brown on the outside and just done in the middle.

RISSOLES

Like prunes in lumpy custard and spam fritters, rissoles were one of those things we used to joke about at school. All I really remember is that they were made with minced beef and rice (I think) – and I'm guessing breadcrumbs. Anyway, this is how I make mine; have them hot with vegetables and a few potato wedges, or cold with salad and pitta bread.

Use whichever kind of rice you like, and instead of beef, minced pork or lamb are also good.

MAKES APPROXIMATELY 10 LARGE RISSOLES:
1lb (450–500 g) mince
6oz (150 g) rice
8oz (200 g) white breadcrumbs
2 eggs, beaten
¼ cup of milk
Seasoning

METHOD
1. Cook rice in the usual way, then strain through a sieve and immediately rinse with plenty of cold water.
2. Mix the beaten eggs with about ¼ cup of milk and spread the breadcrumbs out on a large, shallow tray.
3. Put the cooked rice into a very large bowl with the raw mince (and whatever herbs and spices you want to use) and squish it together gently with your hands.
4. Shape into Scotch egg size balls – or slightly smaller – dip them into the egg mixture, then coat with the breadcrumbs.
5. Heat enough oil in a very large saucepan to just cover the rissoles (a piece of stale bread will turn golden in less than 30 seconds if the oil's hot enough) and deep fry for a few minutes

until the coating is crisp and brown.

6   Put the rissoles on an ovenproof tray in a moderate oven, Gas Mark 4 (180°C) for about 20 minutes.

ALSO TRY...

1.   BEEF & CHEESE CRUMBLE: Make a crumble with 6 oz (150 g) plain flour, 3 oz (75 g) of butter and 1 oz (25 g) of grated cheese for topping a casserole made with a family-sized pack of mince, thoroughly cooked with onions, mushrooms and sweetcorn, then mixed with a thick gravy, seasoning and a dash of Worcester Sauce.

2.   SPAGHETTI BOLOGNESE *(see Chapter 10: Weekly Menu Planning)*.

3.   Use up small amounts of uncooked mince to make tiny meatballs *(see Chapter 4: Quick Fixes)* for mixing with pasta and tomato sauce.

CHICKEN

There's been a never-ending stream of bad publicity regarding chicken and turkey farming in recent years; maybe it's still so popular because, not counting sausages and burgers, children seem to prefer it to any other kind of meat.

I must admit I still love chicken and turkey, and I think as long as you steer well clear of the dodgy stuff – by which I mean chicken from any fast food outlet, the chill cabinet or supermarket freezer, and anything that isn't proven free range (check for the little tractor logo on the packaging) – you should be fairly safe.

Just in case you haven't seen and heard enough hard evidence already about the horror that is cheap chicken, it's usually been farmed and handled in extremely unhygienic conditions, then pumped full of water and chemicals to increase the weight, which means you're paying more money for less (poor quality) meat.

Chicken dishes made from reconstituted meat, including the ones marketed for children, are even worse. Skin, fat, a whole host of other body parts and cheap fillers are just a few of the things you could be swallowing every time you eat chicken Kiev or a slice of turkey roll, and although one of the manufacturers' favourite claims is 'made with 100% breast meat', what they don't tell you is that the product only contains about 56% meat in the first place: low grade, factory farmed and full of water; the rest is batter and breadcrumbs.

CHICKEN NUGGETS

Not to be confused with the sort of nuggets, dippers, drummers or burgers you find in the supermarket; call them what you will, they're all made from the same processed rubbish.

The worst chicken burgers I've ever come cross were the ones in primary school dinners, where they appeared on the menu in a variety of shapes and sizes virtually every day. They were all basically the same; rubbery, too salty and utterly flavourless, except for one type we used to call petrol burgers, because dirty petrol was what they smelt and tasted of.

I came across petrol burgers again a couple of years ago when I bought a chicken burger for one of my children at a health club – more fool me. Needless to say, it was inedible; one bite and the rest went straight into the bin.

But don't give up on chicken nuggets altogether, make them at home instead. These chicken nuggets are made with real free-range chicken fillets and, surprise, surprise; real chicken is exactly what they taste of. Don't be tempted to leave the carrots, apples and onion out; not only do they make the chicken go further, they really do add flavour (and vitamins) and make the nuggets more tender and that bit tastier.

MAKES APPROXIMATELY 20 GOOD-SIZED NUGGETS:
2 free-range chicken fillets
2 large carrots
2 apples
1 large onion
Breadcrumbs, approx 1lb (450–500 g)
2 eggs + milk, beaten together

OPTIONAL:
Flour
Lemon juice
Tarragon or thyme
Salt and pepper

METHOD

1. Wash and roughly chop the carrots and onion, peel and core the apples, remove the skin from the chicken and cut the meat into large pieces.

2. If you're using the above quantities, blend the whole lot in one go in a 2 litre food processor. If you've got a smaller food processor or you're making twice as many nuggets, blend the chicken first, followed by the fruit and vegetables. *Although you can whiz everything to a smooth paste if you like, I prefer my nuggets to have a chunkier texture, so blend the ingredients on a slow setting to get the consistency you want. Alternatively, grate the fruit and vegetables by hand with a cheese grater and snip the chicken into tiny pieces with kitchen scissors.*

3. Put the blended ingredients into a large bowl and squish it all together with your hands, adding some breadcrumbs if you feel the mixture is a bit wet.

4. Spread the breadcrumbs across a large, fairly shallow dish or tray and beat the eggs together in a bowl with approximately 4 fl oz of milk. (Coat the nuggets in flour before dipping them

in the beaten egg mixture if you like; I don't bother.)

5. Shape the nuggets with your hands, dipping each one into the egg mixture first, and working with only a small amount of breadcrumbs at a time to avoid making a mess of the whole tray and creating too much waste.

6. To cook the nuggets: Warm enough oil, about 2 inches (5 cms), in a large pan to completely cover the nuggets and test if it's hot enough by dropping a small chunk of bread into the pan; it should go brown in a matter of seconds. If the oil is too cool the nuggets will break up and go soggy; if it's just right they should turn crisp and golden in about a minute.

7. Fry the nuggets for a few minutes, then place on a baking tray and finish them off in a warm oven, Gas Mark 4 (180°C) for about 15 minutes to cook through. N.B. If you're freezing chicken nuggets, place them side by side (uncooked) on a small tray, cover them with foil and tie them into a freezer bag, or layer them with greaseproof paper in a plastic container and seal tightly with a lid. When you take them out, allow them to thaw slightly for a few minutes so they're easier to separate, remove excess moisture with kitchen roll, and for best results follow the cooking instructions above.

CHICKEN CURRY

If want a meatier curry, double up the amount of chicken and use the same quantity of vegetables.

SERVES 4–6:
At least 4 chicken fillets, skin removed
1 large onion
2 cloves of garlic, crushed
1 medium-sized carrot
Mushrooms

1 small carton of natural yoghurt (or 4 tbsp from a big carton)
½ pint chicken stock (1 stock cube)
Oil
Tomato puree
1 sachet of coconut paste

SPICES:
2 tsp (plus) medium curry powder
1 tsp cumin
½ tsp coriander
½ tsp ginger

METHOD
1. Wash and finely slice the onion, carrot and mushrooms.
2. Remove chicken skin, rinse the meat in cold water, dry well and cut into narrow strips.
3. Warm some oil with the spices and crushed garlic in a very large saucepan and quickly fry the chicken pieces for a couple of minutes.
4. Turn the heat down and add the onion, carrot and mushrooms, making sure everything is coated with the spices.
5. Pour in the stock, followed by the yoghurt and coconut, and stir well.
6. Cover with a lid and cook gently for up to an hour, stirring occasionally, or transfer the curry to a casserole dish with a lid and cook in the oven, Gas Mark 3 (160/170°C) for the same amount of time.
7. Serve with plain boiled rice.

MEXICAN CHICKEN

The Tex Mex seasoning you get with DIY taco kits tends to be made with chilli powder, coriander and cumin, so if you have all these spices in your cupboard already, it's cheaper and more convenient to make your own. (And as a rough guide, I'd say one medium-sized chicken fillet makes two wraps.)

I like those long, thin, sweet red peppers for this, but any peppers will do. (Add a chilli pepper if you like it hot.)

To make 6:

3 Chicken fillets, cut into strips
1 small onion
Tortilla wraps, flour wraps, or taco shells
1 each, small red and green peppers
Oil

For the seasoning:

4 tsp ground cumin
4 tsp ground coriander
1 tsp (plus) medium chilli powder
Salt and pepper

Method

1. Remove chicken skin, wash well and cut the chicken into thin strips.
2. Mix the seasoning together on a dinner plate and coat the meat (you can always make more if you run out) or, if you prefer, add the spices to the hot oil.
3. Heat the oil in a large pan and quickly fry the chicken on the outside.
4. Turn the heat down, add the thinly sliced peppers and onion, and cook for a few minutes until soft.
5. Serve with shredded lettuce and thinly sliced tomato and cucumber in wraps or taco shells, or with plain boiled rice and guacamole.

CHICKEN & HAM PASTA BAKE

This only takes a few minutes longer than a pasta bake made with a jar of instant sauce, and apart from having a far superior flavour it also contains a lot less salt.

If you don't have tomato juice, use two tins of chopped tomatoes or a carton of passata (finely chopped and sieved tomatoes) instead.

I only use two chicken breasts to save money, but there's no reason why you can't use more chicken than this without making any other alterations to the recipe.

SERVES 4 −6:
2 chicken breast fillets (skin removed)
½ packet (say 5 slices) honey roast ham
Mushrooms
1 onion
1 clove of garlic
1 ½ pint (¾ litre) tomato juice
2 big tbsp soft cream cheese (or Quark) or half a tub, approx 8 oz
    (300 g)
Dried pasta shapes (approx 1 handful per person)
2 tsp rosemary (or mixed herbs)
2 handfuls of grated cheese (a mix of mozzarella and cheddar is good)
1 packet of ready salted crisps (scrunched up in the bag)
Olive oil

METHOD
1. Warm a little olive oil in a large saucepan; cut the chicken fillets into strips or small pieces and fry gently with the onion and garlic for a few minutes.
2. Add the mushrooms and ham, followed by the herbs, tomato

juice and cream cheese, stirring for a few minutes until the cheese has blended thoroughly into the tomato sauce.

3. Put the (uncooked) pasta into the pan with the sauce, mix well, then pour the whole lot into a large ovenproof dish, making sure all the pasta is covered.

4. Top with the grated cheese and scrunched up crisps and bake in the oven, Gas Mark 4 (180°C) for 30–40 minutes, by which time the pasta should be perfectly cooked.

SWEET & SOUR CHICKEN

With couscous instead of rice, this is very nearly a quick fix. If you want to make it with pork instead of chicken you'll need to cook the meat a bit longer, simmering for 20 –30 minutes instead of 10, once the sauce has been made.

SERVES 6:
4 chicken fillets
1 red pepper
1 orange or yellow pepper
1 onion
1 standard tin of pineapple rings
2 tbsp vinegar (malt, white, or white wine)
2 tbsp tomato puree
2 tbsp soy sauce
1 rounded tbsp sugar (soft brown or white)
Oil
Plain flour

METHOD
1. Warm some oil in a large saucepan.
2. Remove chicken skin, wash and cut into strips or small pieces

and coat in a little plain flour.

3. Fry the chicken on all sides, then turn the heat right down and cover with a lid while you finely chop the onion and peppers.
4. Add the onion and peppers to the pan; cut 3 or 4 pineapple rings into small pieces and put them in followed by the vinegar, tomato puree, soy sauce, sugar and all the juice from the tin of pineapple.
5. Stir well, cover with a lid and simmer very gently for about 10 minutes.

ALSO TRY:

1. Chicken in Cream & Mushroom Sauce: Coat chicken thighs in a little flour or chicken seasoning (say two pieces of chicken per adult), then fry in butter and olive oil, adding crushed garlic, finely chopped onions and mushrooms, seasoning – mixed herbs, coriander and nutmeg are all good – and a medium-sized tub of single cream. Simmer gently for about 25 minutes while you make boiled rice and a mixed salad.
2. Chicken Goujons: Make chicken fillets into chicken goujons by cutting them into long, thin strips, dunking in beaten egg and breadcrumbs and deep frying, as you would with chicken nuggets.

SAUSAGES

Poor old sausages have come in for a lot of stick in recent years, and let's face it, some of them deserve their bad reputation, especially if the horror stories about what goes into them are to be believed; cows' eyeballs and pigs' snouts are two of the less repulsive ingredients I've heard about.

Sadly, I have to say I do believe the stories – and once again, the worst examples I've come across were in primary school dinners. As a rough guide, go for sausages that contain an absolute minimum of 70% meat, and preferably 80% plus (you'll see from the ingredients listed on the back of the packaging) and don't be tempted by the cheaper ones. It's not worth it.

TOAD IN THE HOLE

Always, *always* use plain flour for Yorkshire pudding – if you use self-raising you'll get a flat, solid result – and make sure the oil is at least *fizzing*, if not *smoking* hot when you pour the batter in; that's the secret of perfect Yorkshire pudding. Some people say you should make the batter in advance and rest it in the fridge for a while, but I don't think it makes a lot of difference. Plain flour and hot oil are the magic ingredients – and use 2 eggs instead of one, even for smaller quantities of Yorkshire pudding; that way your pudding will have more substance and stay firm and well-risen, instead of shrinking up and losing its perfect shape a few seconds after you take it out of the oven.

As a rough guide, use one heaped tablespoon of flour per person and add the milk gradually so you can see where you are with it before you make the batter too thin and have to start sifting in more flour.

SERVES 4:
8 sausages
4 oz (100 g) plain flour
2 eggs
Milk, splash
Oil

OPTIONAL:
1 small onion (finely chopped)

METHOD

1. Arrange the sausages evenly in a large ovenproof dish with some extra oil. (The sausages make their own fat, but you need more to cook the Yorkshire pudding in; an extra 3– 4 tablespoons should do it.) Prick the sausages a few times with a sharp knife and put them in a hot oven, Gas Mark 6/7 (200/220°C). If you're using the onion, chop it finely and scatter around the sausages after about 10–15 minutes when the oil is hot and the sausages are starting to go brown.

2. Now sift the flour in a largish mixing bowl (give yourself plenty of elbow room) and make a well in the centre.

3. Break the eggs into the well, one at a time; add a big splash of milk and start whisking, gradually adding more milk until you've got a fairly thick, smooth, pouring batter. You can leave the batter in the fridge, but have it ready to pour into the very hot oil the minute you bring the sausages from the oven.

4. When the sausages are brown and very nearly done, quickly pour the batter in and return to the top half of the oven immediately. After about 20 minutes you should have lovely dark brown sausages and perfect golden, well-risen Yorkshire pudding.

CIDER SAUSAGES

According to traditional recipes you're meant to cook the sausages in the sauce for part of the time, but I don't see the point unless you like your sausages soft and soggy. I think it works better to do the sausages separately (in the oven, or grill them) and just pour the sauce over them on the plate at the end.

Use mushrooms and sweet red pepper instead of carrots if you prefer, in which case you'll only need to simmer the sauce for about 20 minutes instead of half an hour.

FOR THE CIDER SAUCE:

1 onion

2 celery sticks

2 carrots

2 tbsp plain flour

$^3/_4$ pint (450 ml) medium dry apple cider

$^1/_4$ pint (125 ml) beef stock

Butter

Oil

Parsley

Salt & pepper

1 bouquet garni

METHOD

1. Wash and chop the onion, carrots and celery as thinly as you can; warm the butter and oil in a large saucepan and fry the vegetables until the onion is soft and slightly golden.
2. Stir in 2 tbsp of plain flour and cook for another minute, then add the stock and the cider with the bouquet garni and bring to the boil.
3. Turn the heat right down and simmer for 30–40 minutes, or until the carrots are just soft, adding parsley and seasoning to taste.

ALSO TRY...

1. JAMIE OLIVER-STYLE PAN-FRIED SAUSAGES: Split sausages in half lengthways, open up and fry them flat for cooking in double-quick time.
2. SAUSAGES IN CURRY SAUCE: Use up leftover curry sauce (or a jar of readymade if you're desperate) by re-heating in the microwave and pouring over well-done sausages and plain boiled rice.

PORK

Tips

For the very best crackling, roast a joint of pork with the rind on for the first hour, then remove the rind and cook separately at the top of the oven.

Don't waste time making apple sauce; a large jar of organic baby apple puree does the same job.

SAUSAGE ROLLS

Sausage rolls are usually made with puff pastry; too tricky and time-consuming for most of us to tackle at home, so I make sausage rolls with suet which is dead easy to handle – even for very inexperienced pastry makers – and which, contrary to popular belief, actually contains less saturated fat than butter.

These sausage rolls are especially nice hot (they're perfect with mashed potatoes, green vegetables and gravy), but are also good cold and keep well in the fridge for quite a few days.

MAKES APPROXIMATELY 12 SAUSAGE ROLLS:

FOR THE FILLING:
1 lb (450–500 g) Pork mince
1 large jar of baby apple (or apple & apricot) puree, or 1 tin of apple chunks
1 small sachet of sage & onion stuffing mix

FOR THE PASTRY:
8 oz (225 g) self raising flour
4 oz (100 g) suet
6 fl oz (175 ml) water (approx)

METHOD
1. Combine the pork, stuffing mix and apple chunks (or puree) in a food processor or blender – or squish it all together in a large bowl with your hands.
2. Mix the flour and suet together in a large bowl and gradually add the water to form a ball of dough. The dough should be quite soft, but firm enough to handle easily; if it's too sticky, sprinkle more flour into the mixing bowl and keep kneading it gently until it feels right.
3. Roll the dough out on a floured surface into a large rectangle; as thin as you can get it without tearing.
4. Form the sausage meat into a fat roll, roughly the same length as the pastry, and place in the middle. Fold one side of the pastry across the meat and brush it with milk; bring the opposite side of the pastry over, pressing it down gently to hide the join, then brush the top and sides of the giant sausage roll with milk, trim the rough ends and cut it crossways into slices. You should get about a dozen sausage rolls roughly two inches thick.
5. Place the sausage rolls on an oiled baking tray and bake in the oven for 20–25 minutes, until the pastry is a deep golden brown and the meat is obviously cooked through.

SWEET APPLE & APRICOT PORK

SERVES 4–6:
4 –8 pork fillets
1 red onion
2 small apples
Dried apricots, handful
Oil

FOR THE SAUCE:
½ pint (250 ml) pork or vegetable stock (made with 1 stock cube)
1 tbsp golden syrup
1 tsp butter
1 tsp plain flour
2 tsp sage

METHOD
1. Wash and finely chop the apples, apricots and onion and remove any excess fat from the pork fillets.
2. Warm enough oil to just cover the bottom of a large pan and quick fry the pork fillets with the finely chopped onion, turning once.
3. Place the pork and onion in a large ovenproof dish and cover with the apples and apricots.
4. Blend the flour, butter and sage together in a mixing jug to make a smooth paste; add the stock cube, syrup and ½ pint (250 ml) of boiling water, whisking with a fork or small hand whisk until everything has dissolved.
5. Pour the sauce over the pork and cover the dish with a lid or a sheet of silver foil.
6. Cook in a moderate oven, Gas Mark 4 (180°C) for about an hour, or until the pork is tender.

GINGER BEER PORK

SERVES 4–6:

1 lb (450–500 g) pork fillets
2 tbsp flour
Salt & pepper
½ pint (250 ml) ginger beer
½ pint (250 ml) pork or vegetable stock
1 onion
2tsp brown sugar
1 clove of garlic
1 tsp caraway seeds
Oil

METHOD

1. Warm some oil in a large saucepan while you cut the pork into thin strips and coat lightly in the seasoned flour.
2. Quick fry the pork; strain the old oil if it's a bit dirty and add some fresh to the pan with the onion and garlic.
3. Stir in the stock and the ginger beer with the sugar and caraway seeds; bring to the boil then reduce the heat and simmer very *gently* for 45 minutes –1 hour, until the pork is tender. Serve with any combination of winter vegetables and lots of mashed potato.

SPICY PORK MEATBALLS

The quantities given below make at least 30 tiny meatballs, so if you don't need this many now, freeze some – or cook the lot and put the leftovers in a salad the following day. It's a bit fiddlier making the meatballs this small, but for my money they work better as gobstoppers than ping pong balls.

MAKES 30 TINY MEATBALLS:

1 lb (450–500 g) minced pork

³⁄₄ cup of breadcrumbs

1 large egg

6 tbsp flour (plain or wholemeal plain)

1 tbsp curry powder

1 tbsp cumin

Pepper

METHOD

1. Put the meat in a large bowl and squish it up with the egg and breadcrumbs.
2. Sift the flour and spices onto a large dinner plate.
3. Roll the mixture into balls and coat in the seasoned flour.
4. Shallow fry in very hot oil for 10–15 minutes and serve with a tomato sauce *(see DIY Pasta Sauce later in this chapter and Quick Tomato Sauce in Chapter 10: Weekly Menu Planning)* and either rice or pasta, or mashed potatoes.

ALSO TRY...

1. PORK IN PLUM SAUCE: Quickly brown some pork fillets in a pan, then transfer to a casserole dish, cover with a lid and cook in a moderate oven, Gas Mark 3 (170°C) while you stew 1 lb (500 g) of plums in a saucepan with a little water, 1 level tbsp of soft brown sugar, ½ tsp of cinnamon and ¼ pint of red wine. After 15 minutes when the plums are soft, push them through a sieve, pour the puree over the pork and continue cooking for about 1 hour until the pork is tender.
2. GREEK-STYLE PORK: Cut pork fillets into strips and seal the meat in a large saucepan with very hot oil; cover with a lid and simmer gently for 30–40 minutes, then add half a small bag of torn up spinach, 1 tsp of nutmeg and ½ large carton of natural

yoghurt mixed with 1 tbsp of plain or wholemeal flour; stir well and simmer gently for another 10 minutes. Serve with pitta bread and salad.

BEEF

Tips

Use kitchen scissors for cutting up raw meat; it's much quicker and more hygienic than messing about with knives and chopping boards.

Stir in a spoonful of mustard straight from the jar to give beef dishes an extra kick, or make a casserole with ½ pint (250 ml) of stout instead of beef stock and cook slowly for 1 ½ –2 hours until the meat is tender.

STEAK & KIDNEY PUDDING

Be careful not to flood the pudding when you pour the stock onto the meat; although I've said ¼ pint in the list of ingredients you won't need that much, so add it slowly and carefully. Alternatively, you can mix a crumbly stock cube with the flour you use to coat the meat in at the beginning – Oxo cubes are best – in which case, add plain cold water to the meat instead of stock.

SERVES 6:
FOR THE PASTRY:
½ lb (225 g) self-raising flour
4 oz (100 g) suet (beef or vegetable)
6 fl oz (175 ml) cold water (approx)

FOR THE FILLING:
1 lb (450 – 500 g) stewing steak
¾ lb (375 g) lamb's kidneys
3 tbsp sherry
Worcester sauce
2 tbsp plain flour
Salt & pepper
Mixed herbs
¼ pint (125 ml) beef stock (made with ½ stock cube or 1 tsp Marmite or 1 Oxo cube)

METHOD
1. Trim any excess fat off the meat, wash and dry well, then coat in the seasoned flour and mix with the herbs, sherry, and a dash of Worcester sauce.
2. Make the stock (if you haven't already coated the meat with an Oxo cube) and leave to cool.
3. Make the pastry by sifting the flour into a large bowl with the suet, then adding the cold water and mixing with one hand to form a soft but still fairly stiff dough.
4. Roll the dough out on a floured surface to make a big enough circle to fill a 2 pint (approximately 1 litre) pudding basin (earthenware or Pyrex) with at least an inch (2.5 cm) overlapping, then cut out one quarter of the pastry circle to make the lid.
5. Line the pudding basin with the large piece of pastry, pressing it down to the bottom of the basin and sealing the join with your fingers.
6. Fill the pudding with the meat mixture and approximately 2 fl oz (60 ml) of beef stock or cold water then put the pastry lid on and trim the overlap, leaving just enough to fold over the lid and seal the pudding. (Make it stick by painting a little

water along the edge of the pudding with your fingers first.)

7. Cover the pudding with a double layer of greaseproof paper with a pleat in the middle to allow for the pudding to expand, followed by a piece of foil, also pleated in the middle.

8. Steam the pudding in a large saucepan with a lid on for 3–3 ½ hours, checking the water level in the saucepan every so often to see that it doesn't boil dry.

9. You can serve the pudding straight from the basin, otherwise hold an oven tray firmly over the top and turn the basin over; the pudding should slide out slowly and stay in one perfect piece. Pop the tray into the oven to keep the pudding warm.

BEEF STROGANOFF

Usually made with fillet steak, a cheaper and equally good version can be made with rump or braising steak; all you need to do is cook the meat a bit longer.

SERVES 6:
1 ½ – 2 lb (roughly 1 kg) steak
1 medium onion
½ lb (225 g) button mushrooms
1 teaspoon mustard, preferably Dijon
1 small (5 oz) carton of single cream
2 tbsp sherry or brandy
Parsley
Butter
Oil

METHOD

1. Heat some oil in a large frying pan; cut the steak into fine strips, sprinkle with a little salt and pepper and quick-fry for

a minute to seal the meat on all sides before turning the heat right down and letting steak simmer very gently for about half an hour.

2. Add a good lump of butter to the pan and fry the finely chopped onions until soft and golden, then add the sliced mushrooms and cook for another 2 or 3 minutes.
3. Stir in the mustard with the brandy (or sherry) and cream; warm through very gently (to stop the cream curdling) for 5–10 minutes.
4. Sprinkle with plenty of parsley and serve with plain boiled rice and salad.

ALSO TRY...

1. BEEF CURRY: Make curry with stewing steak instead of chicken (see Chicken Curry), slow-cooking the meat for an extra 15–20 minutes at the start, before you add the vegetables and make the sauce.

LAMB

LANCASHIRE HOT POT

Lancashire hot pot was traditionally made with lamb chops or cutlets on the bone; use them if you like, but I prefer to use neck fillet, which only needs a slightly longer cooking time to become as succulent and juicy as the most expensive leg of lamb. *(See also Scotch Broth in Chapter 5: The Joy of Soup.)*

SERVES 6:
2 lb (1 kg) neck fillet of lamb
2 lb (1 kg) potatoes

1 large onion
1 pint of lamb or beef stock
Oil
Butter
Thyme
Rosemary
Salt & pepper

METHOD

1. Peel the potatoes, rinse them well and slice into rings about ⅛ inch (2mm) thick.
2. Heat some oil in a large pan, fry the onion for a few minutes, then add the lamb and brown the meat quickly on all sides.
3. Put half the potato rings on the bottom of a deep ovenproof dish, cover with the lamb and onions and season well.
4. Pour in the hot stock, then layer the rest of the potatoes on top of the meat and dot with small pieces of butter.
5. Cover the casserole with a lid, or a sheet of foil, and cook in a moderate oven, Gas Mark 4 (180°C) for about 2 hours, then remove the lid and continue cooking for another 15–20 minutes until the potatoes on the top are golden brown and crisp around the edges.

ALSO TRY...

1. KEBABS: If you have meat left over from a joint of lamb, this is the perfect way to enjoy a guilt-free kebab without risking your health and wondering what, exactly, is inside that festering thunder-thigh rotating on the spike in your local kebab shop. Simply re-heat the meat by frying quickly in very hot oil, then turn the heat down, cover with a lid and keep warm while you wash some salad and warm the pitta bread under the grill. Make a great spicy mint sauce by blending the

following ingredients together, in no particular order and mixing with the cooked lamb. (For a thicker sauce just add more yoghurt.):

2 tbsp natural yoghurt
1 tbsp vinegar
1 tsp mint
1 heaped tsp sugar
½ tsp curry powder
½ tsp turmeric
½ tsp salt

2. MEDALLIONS OF LAMB IN RED WINE: Slice approximately 1 ½ lb (600 g) of neck fillet into medallions and brown the meat in a pan with butter and olive oil, adding a finely chopped red onion, mushrooms and half a bottle of red wine, then simmer for about 45 minutes, or until the meat is tender. Thicken the sauce with a little cornflour mixed with a couple of spoonfuls of liquid from the pan, plus a small spoonful each of gravy granules and tomato puree; serve with new potatoes, or mash, and green vegetables.

LIVER

Raw liver is never a pretty sight. Right up there with Brussels sprouts and lumpy custard, it's one of those things that lots of children, not to mention adults, go green at the mere mention of. Not only that, you have to spend at least ten minutes preparing liver before cooking and you run the risk of splattering blood all over the kitchen if you plonk a plateful down too carelessly on the work top. So what then, is the point of liver?

Well, if you can get past the downside, liver is also pretty tasty, versatile, full of protein – and dirt cheap. Lambs' liver is your best bet for an everyday dinner, closely followed by chicken livers. Ox liver and pigs' liver are even cheaper, but they have a stronger, less pleasant flavour – and they remind me of bad school dinners and pet food. At the other end of the scale, calves' liver is tender and delicious, but considerably more expensive, so even though it's my favourite I only buy it occasionally.

If you don't like the idea of eating liver with fava beans and a nice Chianti, try one of the following recipes...

To prepare liver

Put the liver into a colander and give it a good rinse under the cold tap to get rid of most of the blood; now you can see the skin and any other little bits of sinew that need removing much more easily. (As with any other meat, I find it much easier to cut liver up with kitchen scissors.) Coat the pieces in a little seasoned flour and you're ready to go.

CHICKEN LIVER RISOTTO

Add ½ glass of white wine and ½ tsp of cayenne pepper with the stock for extra zing.

SERVES 4–6:
½ lb (250g) chicken livers
4 rashers of back bacon
1 onion
2 peppers
1 courgette
Mushrooms
A handful of spinach
1 clove of garlic

Rice (roughly one handful per person)
Oil
1 pint (500 ml) (approx) chicken stock made with 2 stock cubes
Thyme
Parsley
Paprika

METHOD

1. Wash and chop the onion, garlic, peppers and courgette.
2. Prepare liver in the usual way; snip into small pieces with the bacon and quick fry for a few minutes in a large saucepan with the oil until the bacon is brown and crisp and the liver is done on the outside.
3. Strain off as much of the oil and liquid as you can; warm some more oil in the pan, then add the onion, garlic, peppers and courgette and cook for a few more minutes, until the onion is soft and golden.
4. Wash and drain the rice, mix it well with the meat and vegetables in the saucepan and add the stock with the herbs. (Don't worry too much about any extra liquid; risotto tends to be wetter than most other rice dishes and you can always strain some of the liquid off at the end once the rice is cooked if you think there's too much.)
5. Cover the saucepan with a lid and simmer very gently for about 15 minutes until the rice is just soft, adding the spinach about five minutes before the end. Sprinkle the finished risotto with paprika and season to taste.

ALSO TRY...

1. LIVER, BACON & ONION: *(See Chapter 10: Weekly Menu Planning).*
2. LIVER IN BLACK BEAN SAUCE: Prepare and pan fry 1 or 2 packets of lambs' liver with a sliced red onion, then add a small

tin of pineapple chunks (without the juice) and the black bean sauce; stir well and simmer for about 15 minutes.

3. SPICY LIVER & PORK MEATBALLS: Add 1 small packet (say 80p worth) of roughly chopped liver to about 1 lb (450 g) of minced pork (*see Spicy Pork Meatballs, in this chapter*).

4. MIXED GRILL: A great favourite back in the 1970s when prawn cocktails and Black Forest Gateau were the height of fashion, a mixed grill is traditionally a fat and cholesterol-laden time bomb. Make a slightly less lethal version by washing and preparing the liver in the usual way, then frying in a little olive oil and butter with some kidney, mushrooms and a small, finely sliced onion. Garnish with watercress and serve with good quality, oven-cooked sausages, grilled tomatoes and potato wedges or oven chips.

FISH

Support your local fishmonger – or the fresh fish counter in your local supermarket, if you're lucky enough to have one. I think lots of us tend to be unadventurous when it comes to buying and cooking fish simply because we just don't know what to do with it and are too shy to ask. British fish stocks have been in crisis for a long time and by now we should all be eating more 'sustainable' fish, such as herrings, sprats, sole, sardines and red mullet. So don't ignore those friendly, helpful faces behind the fish counter any longer; ask for advice and start cooking more fish from this moment on. I will if you will.

Tips

Prawns can be defrosted much more quickly than the instructions on the packaging suggest if you're using them for cooking. Just put them in a colander and rinse well in cold water; leave to drain for about 15 minutes, then rinse well again.

TUNA LASAGNE

If you like, use grated cheddar instead – although cottage cheese makes this a very low fat option – and leave out the parmesan and breadcrumb topping.

Serve with salad, broccoli or any other green vegetables, and extra sweetcorn.

SERVES 4 – 6:
1 tin of tuna (any size)
2 standard tins of chopped tomatoes
Frozen prawns (1 small bag or half a large one)
Spinach (a couple of handfuls)
Frozen sweetcorn (or one small tin)
Lasagne sheets (approx 9)
Lemon juice
Basil
Black pepper

FOR THE CHEESE SAUCE:
1 small carton of cottage cheese
2 oz (50 g) butter
2 oz (50 g) flour
1 pint (500 ml) milk

OPTIONAL:
Parmesan cheese
Breadcrumbs

METHOD

1. Wash the spinach, tear into pieces; drain the tin of tuna and mix with the defrosted prawns, chopped tomatoes, sweetcorn, lemon juice and seasoning in a large bowl.

TO MAKE THE CHEESE SAUCE:

a. Melt the butter in a large saucepan, stir in the flour and cook for a minute until the paste is glazed and shiny looking.

b. Remove from the heat, add the milk and cheese, and return to the heat. Keep stirring the sauce continuously and make it easy on yourself by using a small hand whisk instead of a wooden spoon to stop it going lumpy. (If you want the sauce a bit thinner, just whisk in more milk.)

2. Layer the tuna mixture and the pasta sheets with a couple of spoonfuls of cheese sauce, finishing with a complete layer of cheese sauce on the top.

3. Sprinkle the breadcrumbs and grated parmesan and bake in a moderate oven, Gas Mark 4 (180°C) for 20–30 minutes until the sauce is bubbling and the top is a deep golden brown.

SWEET & SPICY PRAWNS

SERVES 4–6:

1 large bag of frozen prawns, defrosted
2 red or orange peppers
1 small tin of baby sweetcorn
3 –4 broccoli florets
2 tbsp soft brown sugar
¼ pint (125 ml) hot water

1 level teaspoon chilli powder
Soy sauce
Garlic puree
Tomato puree
Sesame seeds
Olive oil
2–3 shredded wheat style squares of dried noodles

METHOD
1. Defrost the prawns *(see tips page 76)*.
2. Heat the oil in a wok or very large saucepan; cut peppers into thin strips, slice the baby sweetcorn whichever way you want and chop the broccoli into tiny florets.
3. Stir fry the vegetables in the hot oil for a few minutes with the sesame seeds.
4. Meanwhile, dissolve 2 tbsp soft brown sugar, 1 tbsp each of tomato and garlic puree in ¼ pint (125 ml) of boiling water, add the soy sauce and chilli powder and mix well.
5. Pour the liquid into the pan, turn up the heat, add the prawns and cook for another few minutes until everything is hot and the vegetables are just tender.
6. Break the dried noodles up a bit and add at the same time as the prawns, otherwise leave the noodles out altogether and cook some white long grain rice instead.

KEDGEREE

Kedgeree is traditionally a breakfast dish, but there can't be many people who can eat this much food first thing in the morning.

Use whichever type of rice you like; I use brown rice and add sesame seeds to give it a nice, nutty flavour – and this is yet another dish you could easily sneak spinach into if you wanted.

Kedgeree may sound unexciting at best and pretty revolting at worst, but it's actually lovely, tasty and warmly satisfying; hopefully even your kids will like it. Over the years I've perfected my technique to the point where the whole thing takes less than half an hour and makes hardly any washing up. What more could you ask for?

SERVES 4–6:
Brown rice (about 1 handful per person)
Smoked mackerel
3 –4 hard boiled eggs
Sesame seeds
3 or 4 spring onions (or 1 regular onion)
1 clove of garlic
Small handful of frozen peas
Oil
Butter
$\frac{1}{2}$ tsp curry powder
Parsley
Lemon juice

METHOD
1. Put the rice in a large saucepan of fresh, slightly salted water, stir, pop the eggs in and put the pan on the stove over a high heat.
2. Bring to the boil; boil rapidly for a minute, then turn the heat down low and cover with a lid.
3. Meanwhile, prepare the smoked mackerel by removing the skin and checking carefully for bones; flake the fish in a bowl, then peel and finely chop the onions.
4. After the eggs have boiled with the rice for about ten minutes, remove them from the saucepan with a slotted spoon, put them to one side and add the frozen peas to the boiling water.

Turn the heat up until the water's boiling again, then turn it down and let it simmer for about 5 minutes, or until the rice is ready. (Don't let the rice overcook and go soggy.)

5. While you're waiting for the rice, peel the hard boiled eggs and chop them into chunks. Warm the oil in a large pan or a wok.

6. Strain the cooked rice and peas through a colander and pour freshly boiled water from the kettle through the colander to remove any trace of starch; add a lump of butter to the rice in the colander and gently stir it in.

7. Fry the onion, sesame seeds and curry powder in the warm oil until the onion starts to soften, then add the fish and cook for another minute or two.

8. Add the rice and peas, hard boiled eggs and plenty of parsley, mix well and when you're sure it's warm enough, sprinkle with lemon juice and serve.

FISHCAKES

MAKES 12 LARGE FISH CAKES:
4 fairly large potatoes
6 frozen skinless cod fillets
1 medium-sized tin of tuna
Lemon juice
Butter
Milk
Black pepper
½ lb (225 g) breadcrumbs, approx
1 small tin of sweetcorn

METHOD
1. Cook the frozen cod fillets in an ovenproof dish, according to the instructions on the packet (this usually takes between

15–20 minutes).

2. Meanwhile, boil the potatoes – with or without the skins – before mashing them with a tablespoonful of butter and some milk.

3. Use a slotted spoon to transfer the fish to a mixing bowl and flake with a fork, then drain the tins of tuna and sweetcorn and add them to the bowl with lots of lemon juice and black pepper.

4. Add the mashed potatoes to the bowl, mix well, then form into fishcakes with your hands.

5. Gently press the fishcakes into a tray of breadcrumbs on both sides (you don't have to dip them into beaten egg unless you want to) and fry in a large saucepan for a few minutes, with enough hot oil to completely submerge the fishcakes. Keep warm in the oven and serve with chips or potato wedges and green vegetables or salad.

ALSO TRY...

1. FASTEST-EVER FISH CAKES: *(see Chapter 4: Quick Fixes)*.

2. FISH PIE: Use a mixture of white fish, tinned tuna, and prawns mixed with lemon juice, seasoning, ½ glass of white wine and a basic cheese sauce made with 2 tbsp flour, 2 oz (50 g) butter, ½ pint (250 ml) of milk and 2 oz (50 g) of grated cheddar cheese; top with mashed potato and cook in the oven for 20 minutes, until the potato browns and the sauce bubbles.

3. GRILLED SARDINES: Melt 2 oz (50 g) of butter in a saucepan and stir in 1 teaspoon each of coriander, paprika, sugar and Tabasco sauce; make a series of diagonal cuts on both sides of the fish from head to tail, coat the fish and grill for about 5 minutes on each side, turning once.

(MOSTLY) VEGETARIAN

Tips

Use aluminium foil *shiny side inwards* to direct more heat towards the food.

Eat shoots and leaves; packets of mixed stir fry vegetables are good value and you can add extra mushrooms, peppers, bean sprouts or onions according to taste.

STUFFED PEPPERS

Life may be too short to stuff a mushroom, as Shirley Conran famously said, but it's definitely not too short to stuff peppers. If you're using very large peppers you'll probably only need one each, otherwise make it two small peppers per person.

SERVES 4–6:
4 large bell peppers, mixed colours
1 packet of Quorn pieces
1 onion or a few shallots
4–6 mushrooms
2 cloves of garlic
1 tsp mixed spice
1 tsp cumin
1 large mugful, approx 8 oz (225 g) couscous
Butter
Olive oil

OPTIONAL:
1 vegetable stock cube
Grated cheese

METHOD

1. Slice the tops off the peppers, get rid of the stalks and wash the tops and the whole peppers inside and out. Stand the peppers up in a deep roasting pan and pre-heat the oven to about Gas Mark 6 (200°C).
2. Finely chop the onions, mushrooms and tops of the peppers and fry in a large pan with butter and olive oil. Add the garlic, about a teaspoon of cumin and the same amount of mixed spice and give it a good stir.
3. Meanwhile, add the boiling water to the couscous in a large bowl (according to the instructions on the packet), stir and leave for a few minutes.
4. Now add the Quorn to the pan with the vegetables, and if you want more liquid, crumble in the stock cube and add a drop of water.
5. Fluff the couscous up with a fork and mix with the vegetables and Quorn.
6. Stuff the peppers, piling any remaining mixture loosely around the base. Cover loosely with foil *(see notes)*, bake in the oven for 20–30 minutes, removing the foil for the last 5 minutes and sprinkling the peppers with grated cheese.

STUFFED MUSHROOMS

On second thoughts, stuffed mushrooms make a great starter or side dish and go very well with rice and salad...

1–2 large flat cap mushrooms per person
White breadcrumbs, a couple of handfuls
Goats' cheese, a couple of ounces
Dried parmesan cheese
Garlic puree
Marmite or Vegemite
Oil
Butter
Parsley

METHOD

1. Remove the stalks then wash and peel the mushrooms – or don't peel and wash the mushrooms; peel but don't wash, or wash but don't peel ... some people say you should, some say you shouldn't. (For what it's worth, I usually do both.)
2. Dissolve a heaped tsp of Marmite or Vegemite (or use a stock cube if you haven't got either) in a small saucepan of boiling water, and poach the mushrooms for a few minutes.
3. Put the warm mushrooms on a grill tray, spread each one with a spoonful of garlic puree topped with crumbly goats' cheese and a mixture of breadcrumbs and parmesan cheese; drizzle with olive oil and grill for a few minutes until the toppings are crusty and brown.

VEGGIE BURGERS

You don't really need an egg to bind the mixture together, but put one in if you like, or used a beaten egg mixed with melted butter to glaze the burgers, instead of oil. Use whatever spices you like – coriander, cayenne pepper and curry powder are all good. Normally, I'm against the idea of smothering food in tomato ketchup, but veggie burgers are one of the few things that really do taste better with lots of it.

MAKES 6 – 8 BURGERS (DEPENDING ON SIZE):
1 tin of chick peas
1 courgette
2 onions
2 carrots
6 tbsp porridge oats
2 cloves of garlic
Thyme
Salt & pepper
Tomato puree
Vegemite
Olive oil
Wholemeal flour

OPTIONAL:
1 egg to bind

METHOD
1. Finely chop the onion; grate the carrots and courgette.
2. Warm some oil in a pan; fry the onion, carrots and courgette over a medium heat and add the crushed garlic and thyme.
3. Meanwhile, drain the chick peas and mash them up a bit with a fork in a large bowl.
4. Put the porridge oats in the bowl with the chick peas, and as soon as the vegetables have softened, throw them in as well.
5. Add a couple of squirts of tomato puree, salt and pepper and 2 tbsp olive oil and mix it all together.
6. Shape the mixture into burgers using your hands and the wholemeal flour and place on an oiled baking tray. Brush the burgers liberally with more oil and bake them in the oven, Gas Mark 6 (200°C) for about 15 minutes.

AUBERGINE LASAGNE

To make a lasagne for more than six people, increase the amount of onion and aubergines and make the cheese sauce with 3 oz each of butter and flour and 1¾ pints of milk. (You don't need to increase the amount of cheese; a little goes a long way.)

Alternatively, make an aubergine bake by omitting the lasagne sheets and using one tin of tomatoes instead of two.

Serve on its own, or with extra green vegetables, sweetcorn, or a mixed salad.

SERVES 4 – 6:
6 – 9 lasagne sheets
1 large or two smaller aubergines
1 onion
2 cloves of garlic, crushed
2 standard size tins of chopped tomatoes
¼ pint (125 ml) vegetable stock
Oil

FOR THE CHEESE SAUCE:
2 oz (50 g) butter or margarine
2 oz (50 g) plain flour
1 pint (500 ml) milk
1 oz (25 g) cheese

OPTIONAL:
¼ bulb of fennel
Parsley

METHOD

1. Wash and thinly slice the aubergines, cut the slices in half and put them in a bowl of salty water *(see notes, page 16)*.
2. Slice or chop the onion and fennel and fry in the oil with the crushed garlic and a good sprinkling of parsley.
3. Add the tinned tomatoes to the pan; bring to the boil and simmer gently while you fry the aubergines.
4. Heat more oil in another pan and to save time fry the aubergine slices on one side only, then drain them on kitchen roll.

To make the cheese sauce:

a. Melt the butter in a large saucepan, stir in the flour and cook for a minute until the paste is glazed and shiny looking.
b. Remove from the heat, add the milk and cheese, and return to the heat. Keep stirring the sauce continuously and make it easy on yourself by using a small hand whisk instead of a wooden spoon to stop it going lumpy. (If you want the sauce a bit thinner, just whisk in more milk.)
5. Layer the lasagne sheets, tomato sauce, aubergines and cheese sauce in a large ovenproof dish, finishing with a layer of cheese sauce on the top, and bake in the oven, Gas Mark 6 (200°C) for 15–20 minutes.

LENTIL MOUSSAKA

SERVES 6:

8 oz (225 g) green lentils or mung beans
1 14 oz (410 g) tin of chopped tomatoes
1 onion, finely chopped
2 cloves of garlic
2 aubergines
Mushrooms (6 – 8 depending on size)
4 medium-large potatoes

1 pint vegetable stock
Oil: sunflower/olive
2 tsp marmite or vegemite
2 tsp basil
1 tsp all spice
Tomato puree

FOR THE TOPPING:
1 pint (500 ml) warm milk
4 oz (100 g) butter
3 tbsp plain flour
2 egg yolks

METHOD

1. Heat a couple of tablespoons of olive oil in a very large saucepan; add the finely chopped onion and garlic and cook for a few minutes until the onion is browning.
2. Add the lentils, chopped tomatoes and stock with the herbs and spices and bring to the boil.
3. Boil quite rapidly for about 5 minutes, then turn the heat down and simmer very gently for about 1 hour until the lentils are soft and mushy.
4. Meanwhile, peel and put the potatoes on to boil in a pan of fresh cold water.
5. Cut the aubergines into thinly sliced quarters and soak in a bowl of cold salty water for 5 minutes while you peel and finely slice the mushrooms.
6. Drain the aubergines thoroughly with kitchen roll, or a clean, dry tea towel, then deep fry in very hot oil.
7. Put the fried aubergines in a bowl and mix with the sliced mushrooms. (The aubergines absorb so much oil there's no need to fry the mushrooms as well.)

8. Slice the boiled potatoes and add about half a tube of tomato puree to the lentils and stir well.
9. Layer the lentil mixture with the aubergines and mushrooms in a large ovenproof dish and finish with a layer of sliced potato.
10. To make the topping, melt the butter in a saucepan and warm the milk – either in another saucepan, or in a large bowl in the microwave (approx 4 minutes on high).
11. Add the flour to the melted butter and stir over the heat for a minute, then pour in the warm milk, whisking all the time.
12. When the sauce starts to thicken, add the egg yolks and whisk for another minute.
13. Pour the topping over the moussaka and bake in the oven for 30 –40 minutes, Gas Mark 4 (180°C) until the sauce is bubbling and the topping has a golden crust.

RICE SALAD

Use whichever type of rice you like, but I think the lighter, fluffier texture of basmati rice is better suited to rice salad than brown or short grain.

Change the salad ingredients around to suit yourself and add some good, diced chicken, ham, prawns, flaked tuna or smoked salmon – this is another good meal for using up leftover bits and pieces.

In fact, there's only one thing you need to be absolutely certain of – as with any dish containing cold rice – and that's making sure you cook and keep it in the right conditions. Because of the starch, warm rice is a haven for the sort of bacteria that can lead to a very nasty stomach upset – or worse.

To avoid trouble, strain the cooked rice in a colander then immediately rinse under cold running water for a minute; absorb the excess moisture with plenty of kitchen roll, and if you're keeping it for later, get the rice covered and into the fridge as quickly as possible. If you're cooking a lot of rice and you only want to save some of it, separate the rice you're planning to keep and follow the above procedure – just don't leave it sitting around in the kitchen for any length of time.

Finally, if you want to warm up cold rice, do it thoroughly, preferably in a pan with very hot oil, until it's piping hot.

½ lb (225 g) basmati rice
Sugar snap peas
Baby sweetcorn
Baby plum tomatoes
Leftover chicken breast meat
A few slices of cold ham
1 avocado
2 spring onions
Chives
Olive oil
Salt & pepper

METHOD
1. Cook the rice in a saucepan of boiling water, boiling rapidly for a couple of minutes, then turn the heat down low and simmer gently for about 10 minutes (don't walk away and do something else; you don't want it mushy and over-cooked).
2. Strain the cooked rice through a colander; rinse with plenty of cold water, remove excess water with kitchen roll, put the rice in a large bowl and cover loosely with a clean cloth or a sheet of foil. (No need to keep it in the fridge if you're planning to eat it straight away; rice salad is one of those things that tastes better at room temperature than it does chilled.)
3. Just cook the baby sweetcorn and sugar snap peas (preferably in the microwave) so they still have plenty of crunch, and add to the rice.

4. Chop the meat, halve the avocado and cut into chunks, then add everything to the bowl of rice with the seasoning, whichever herbs you want to use and a little olive oil.
5. Stir gently, blending everything together without turning it to mush, and serve.

NUT-FREE NUT ROAST

This is more or less the same as the Curried Nut Roast *(see Chapter 10: Weekly Menu Planning)*. If you can't find a bag of mixed seeds in the supermarkets, buy smaller packets and mix them up yourself.

SERVES 6–10:
½ lb (225 g) mixed sunflower, pumpkin and sesame seeds
2 smallish peppers – red/orange and green
1 large onion
1 clove of garlic
1 tin of chick peas
1 carrot, grated
Breadcrumbs made with 4–5 slices of white bread
2 rounded tsp curry powder
1 rounded tsp coriander
Tomato puree
2 eggs, beaten
Olive oil
Sunflower/corn oil

METHOD
1. Make the breadcrumbs in a blender or food processor, then put them in a very large mixing bowl.
2. Blend the seeds and chick peas for about half a minute and add them to the bowl.

3. Meanwhile, chop the onion and peppers and fry with the crushed garlic in a mixture of olive oil and sunflower, or corn oil, until the onion is crisp and golden.
4. Add the fried vegetables to the bowl with the grated carrot, curry powder, coriander, 1 tbsp of tomato puree and the beaten eggs and mix thoroughly – use a fork, it's easier – to bind everything together.
5. Press the mixture into a well greased, standard-sized loaf tin (long-strip-lined with greaseproof paper, see *Lining the tin, page 166*) and bake in a pre-heated oven, Gas Mark 6 (200°C) for about half an hour, until golden.

PIZZA

Contrary to what you may think if you've never made pizza dough before, this is as easy as falling off a log. True, you have to wait a little while for the dough to prove, but so what? If I make pizza I usually do it on a Saturday afternoon so we can eat it in front of the telly in the evening, so pick a time when you don't have to rush off anywhere else for a few hours.

As with most recipes where you get to play with dough, the whole process is a lot of fun and the results are at least as good as anything you get from a pizza parlour, let alone a supermarket.

If you've got enough pans (or 7″ sandwich cake tins) and plenty of oven space you can make individual round pizzas, but I make mine in the same standard-size rectangular oven trays I'd use for a Swiss roll *(see notes, page 196)* and cut them up into squares; usually six large pieces per tray.

THE QUANTITY BELOW MAKES ENOUGH FOR TWO LARGE, THIN & CRISPY TYPE PIZZAS AND ONE SMALL ROUND ONE (SEE ABOVE) – OR TWO LARGE PIZZAS AND 12 DOUGH BALLS.

To make the dough:

1 lb (550 g) plain flour
2 tsp (or 1 sachet) of dried yeast
1 tsp salt
1 tsp sugar
½ pint (250 ml) warm water mixed with 2 tsp oil

Method

1. Mix the dry ingredients together in a large bowl and make a well in the centre.
2. Pour the warm water and oil into the well and quickly mix everything together with your hand to make a soft dough, then turn the dough onto a floured surface and knead it well for a good 5 minutes, sprinkling more flour whenever you feel you need to.
3. Place the dough on a large, greased ovenproof dish, cover with a damp tea towel and leave at the bottom of the oven on the lowest setting for about half an hour, until the dough has swollen and doubled in size.
4. Place the dough on a floured surface and knead it again for another 5 minutes (known as 'knocking back').
5. Put the dough back in the oven to prove again, covered with the damp cloth (which you'll probably need to wet and wring out again) for about half an hour – same as before – until it's doubled in size, then knead the dough again for roughly 5 minutes.
6. Divide the dough into however many pieces you think you're going to need and roll out each piece to more or less the right size and shape for the pan you're using. Gently press the dough into the oiled pan, trim any rough edges and brush the entire surface of the dough with a little more oil. Cover with clingfilm and keep in the fridge until you've got all your bases ready and prepared the toppings, and your pizza is ready to go

in the oven. N.B. *If you have enough dough left over, put it back in the oven covered with the damp cloth for another half an hour, then knead it again and either make another pizza, or wrap it in plenty of clingfilm and put it in the freezer. Alternatively, use leftover dough to make dough balls; just form the dough into ping-pong sized balls, place on a greased tray at the bottom of the oven and serve with garlic butter.*

To make the pizza toppings:
Anything goes really. I usually make one vegetarian and one meaty pizza on the oven trays and mix whatever I've got left over to make the small round pizza, which goes something like this:
Any or all of the following:

2 –3 slices of ham
2 rashers of bacon
Leftover sausages (cooked) or frankfurters
Leftover meatballs
Leftover Bolognese or chilli

1 onion
Green and red pepper
Mushrooms
Spinach
Tomato
Sweetcorn

1 bag of grated mozzarella cheese
Tomato puree
Mixed herbs
Cayenne pepper

METHOD

1. Fry the onion and peppers and divide between two bowls; one meat, one veggie.
2. Fry the mushrooms and spinach, drain a small tin of sweetcorn and add to the veggie bowl.
3. Chop up the leftover sausages, ham, etc and add to the meat bowl.
4. Thinly spread all pizza bases with tomato puree, add the toppings, cover liberally with the grated mozzarella, top with sliced tomato, sprinkle with herbs and spices and bake in a hot oven, Gas Mark 6 – 7 (200/220°C) for about 20 minutes, changing the trays over from top to bottom about halfway through the cooking time.

BAKED POTATO PIZZAS

Eternally popular, it's pizza again; this time on a potato base. *(See also Bread Roll Pizzas, Chapter 10: Weekly Menu Planning.)*

Use the largest baking potatoes you can get; one half should be more than enough for most children (and some adults). Cut the potatoes in half first to reduce the cooking time; prick each potato several times with a sharp knife then either wrap each half in foil and bake in the oven or start them off in the microwave by putting them cut side down on a plate and cooking on high for a few minutes before wrapping in foil and finishing in the oven.

Largest baking potatoes
Grated cheese: a mixture of mozzarella and cheddar is good
Chopped tomatoes
Spring onions
1 red or orange pepper
1 small tin of sweetcorn
Butter

Parsley
Chives
Salt & pepper

METHOD
1. Bake the potatoes in the usual way, then scoop out as much of the soft inside as you can without tearing the skin and causing a total collapse.
2. Put the mashed potato into a bowl with the chopped peppers and onion, sweetcorn, herbs, a couple of tablespoons of chopped tomatoes, some butter and half the grated cheese and mix it all together.
3. Stuff the potato skins with the filling, top with the remainder of the grated cheese and bake the potato pizzas in a moderate oven, Gas Mark 4 (180°C), for about 20 minutes until the pizzas are warmed through and the cheese is brown and bubbly.

CHEESE & ONION TOMATOES

Cheese & onion pie without the pastry; these are great with sausages or bacon and beans for dinner, or as a very filling weekend breakfast. You don't have to feel guilty about discarding the insides of the tomatoes either; keep them in a sealed container in the fridge for a few days and use them up in any recipe that includes chopped tomatoes; chilli, lasagne, shepherd's pie or a pasta sauce.

SERVES 4:
4 large beef tomatoes
2 oz (50 g) grated cheese
2 oz (50 g) breadcrumbs
¼ pint (125 ml) milk

2 eggs, beaten
½ very finely chopped onion
1 tsp plain flour
Salt & pepper

METHOD

1. Cut a circle out of the top of each tomato with a very sharp knife; big enough to enable you to get the knife inside.
2. Discard the tops and use the knife to scrape out some of the tomato to make a hole big enough to fill.
3. Finely chop the onion and coat with the seasoned flour, then mix the onion in a bowl with the breadcrumbs, grated cheese, milk and beaten eggs.
4. Put the tomatoes in an ovenproof dish and spoon the mixture into each one (the amounts given here are enough to fill four beef tomatoes to the top) and bake in the oven, Gas Mark 6 (200°C) for about 30 minutes until the tops are firm and golden.

VEGETABLES

If you only buy fruit and vegetables in season, you'll never be disappointed. (It's not that difficult either when you think about it.) What's the point of eating apricots and plums in January if they taste like polystyrene? And there's nothing to beat British strawberries from the beginning of June till the end of July, so try and resist those bright orangey-red imports you find in the shops all year round; most of the time they're as hard as bullets and taste of nothing.

Tips

Ripen avocados by putting them in a brown paper bag with a banana for a few hours. Also ripen mangoes in a paper bag (without the banana).

For perfect roast potatoes: King Edwards or Maris Pipers are best. Always par boil the potatoes first, simmering for no more than five minutes while you heat the fat in a large ovenproof dish. Strain the water off and bash the potatoes up a bit by shaking them two or three times in the saucepan with the lid on so they're soft enough on the outside to absorb some of the hot fat, which is what makes them lovely and crisp.

Poach mushrooms in Marmite stock instead of frying in butter when you want to cut calories.

Cook all your vegetables in one large saucepan; put the carrots in first (in cold water), then add broccoli or cauliflower with peas or sweetcorn, which only need 3 or 4 minutes, when the carrots are half-cooked. Or buy a vegetable steamer, which makes it easier not to overcook vegetables.

Make gravy by adding the vegetable water to the gravy granules, for extra vitamins.

DIY PASTA SAUCE

Like ratatouille (see below), this pasta sauce is miles better than any of the bottled ones you find in the supermarket. Make it in larger quantities whenever you can so you've got some left over to freeze for another time. (The quantities below make enough for a main meal – with pasta – for about six people.)

DIY Pasta sauce is very versatile, so try these alternatives, or make up your own:

Add a dash of balsamic vinegar or a pinch of cayenne pepper for a spicier flavour.

For a creamy pasta sauce, stir a small carton of soft cream cheese, Quark, or crème fraiche into the sauce at the end.

1 standard tin of plum or chopped tomatoes
2 onions
2 courgettes
Two peppers (any combination of red, green, orange or yellow)
Mushrooms
Spinach (about half a bag)
2 cloves of garlic, crushed
1 vegetable stock cube
Oregano or Italian herbs
Basil
Tomato puree
$^1/_2$ glass of red wine
Olive oil
Butter

METHOD

1. Gently warm butter and oil in a very large pan while you wash and chop the vegetables the way you like them. (If you're planning to blitz the finished sauce in a blender, don't bother fine chopping, just hack it to bits.)
2. Put the garlic and all the vegetables, except the spinach, into the pan, cook for a few minutes until soft, then crumble the stock cube in with the herbs, add the tinned tomatoes and spinach and give it all a good stir.
3. Turn the heat up and let the sauce sizzle before adding the red wine and tomato puree. If you think the sauce is too watery after a couple of minutes, reduce it by keeping the heat up high until the excess liquid evaporates, then turn it down and simmer very gently for a few minutes. To thin the sauce, add more vegetable stock and/or red wine.

RATATOUILLE

SERVES 6 AS AN ACCOMPANIMENT TO A MAIN MEAL:

1 aubergine
2 courgettes
1 onion
1 red pepper
1 green pepper
2 cloves of garlic
2 standard tins of chopped tomatoes
Tomato puree
Basil
Mixed herbs
Olive oil

METHOD

1. Heat olive oil in a very large saucepan; add the onion and crushed garlic and cook gently for about 5 minutes.
2. Meanwhile, top and tail the aubergine and courgettes; slice thinly into rounds, halves or quarters, then soak the aubergine in a bowl of salty water for a few minutes before draining well on plenty of kitchen roll.
3. Dice the red and green peppers and put all the vegetables in the pan with the herbs, chopped tomatoes and a little more olive oil.
4. Give it all a good stir, bring to the boil, then turn the heat right down, adjust the seasoning and add however much tomato puree you think it needs.

ALSO TRY...

1. SKINNY MASH: Don't peel potatoes; just give them a quick wash with a nailbrush in cold water, then boil and mash them in their skins. Known as skinny mash in our house, it saves a lot of time and is much, much nicer than it sounds.

2. BROCCOLI CHEESE: Make cauliflower cheese with broccoli instead of cauliflower, or a combination of both, and serve with pasta, crispy bacon and grilled tomatoes.

3. HONEY & GINGER GLAZED CARROTS: Fry ½ lb (225 g) of thinly sliced carrots in some butter for a few minutes; add a mug of ginger beer and 2 teaspoons each of honey and brown sugar, bring to the boil and simmer for a few minutes until the carrots are just soft.

4. ROASTED VEGETABLES: Any combination of mushrooms, onions or shallots, squash, peppers and finely sliced carrots sprinkled with sesame seeds, basted in olive oil and roasted in a large ovenproof dish for about half an hour.

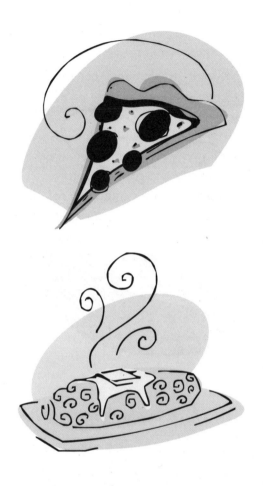

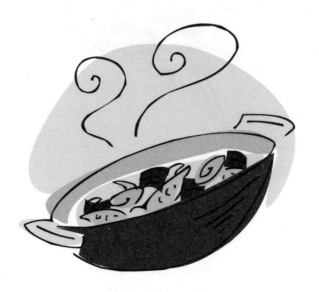

'We may find in the long run that
tinned food is a deadlier weapon
than the machine-gun.'

George Orwell

Quick fixes

The ultimate in speed and simplicity; to qualify as a quick fix a recipe should take no longer than 20 minutes from fridge to table...

Tips

Make a stop-gap version of tomato ketchup with 2–3 tablespoons of tomato puree, 2 teaspoons vinegar, 1 teaspoon of brown sugar and ¼ pint (150ml) of boiling water. (Should be enough for four people.)

To make cold, hard butter straight from the fridge 'spreadable', pop it in the microwave on 'defrost' for about 40 seconds.

For a crunchy, low calorie snack, wash half a bag of curly kale in cold water, sprinkle with salt & vinegar (or any other seasoning you like) and pop into a hot oven on a baking tray for approx 10 minutes.

For chips that taste fried without the hassle of frying (and less calories), drizzle oven chips with a little oil and give them a good shake before you put them in the oven, then again halfway through the cooking time. (Or spice them up by mixing a tablespoon of curry paste or pesto with some hot oil on a large ovenproof tray first.)

Look out for tips and recipe ideas on packaging; you'll find them on everything from lentils, ready-made soups and sauces to packets of biscuits, tinned fruit and jelly.

Freeze wine that's past its best (assuming you ever have any) in an ice cube tray or freezer bag to be popped straight into soups and casseroles when you need them.

QUORN STIR FRY

Obviously a wok is the best thing for a stir fry, but if you don't have one, a very large saucepan or deep-sided frying pan will do. The most important thing with stir fries is to get the meat and vegetables more or less the same size, so everything is ready at the same time, staying crisp and firm, as opposed to ending up a soggy mess.

As for the noodles; use fresh ones if you like, but because they seem fatty and sticky and remind me of tape worms, I prefer the dried ones that come in lumps and look a bit like shredded wheat. (They also keep for at least a year in the cupboard.)

If you've got time, egg fried rice is perfect with this.

SERVES 4:
1 pack Quorn pieces
1 pack stir fry vegetables and bean sprouts
Fine dried noodles (say 4 lumps)
Lime juice
Soy sauce
2 tsp ginger
$\frac{1}{2}$ tsp mixed spice
Sunflower or sesame oil

METHOD
1. Warm the oil in a wok or large deep-sided pan, add the Quorn and turn the heat up.
2. Now add the vegetables and shake vigorously... or just keep turning with a wooden spoon. Add the soy sauce, plenty of lime juice and a couple of teaspoons of ginger.
3. Meanwhile, break up the dried noodles into a bowl of boiling water and leave them to soften and separate; this doesn't take longer than a couple of minutes, so don't overdo.

4. Strain the noodles and add to the pan, stirring occasionally for a couple of minutes, then serve.

PACIFIC PIE

Everyone seems to have their own version of Pacific Pie, so feel free to adapt the basic recipe – a couple of tins of tuna, some kind of sauce and plenty of crisps – to suit yourself. However you make it, it shouldn't take longer than five minutes at a snail's pace.

SERVES APPROXIMATELY 4:
2 large tins of tuna
1 small tin of sweetcorn
1 standard tin of chopped tomatoes
Broccoli
Natural yoghurt
Lemon juice
Grated cheese (Red Leicester is perfect, but cheddar or mozzarella will do)
Ready salted crisps (2 bags)
Black or white pepper

METHOD
1. Wash and break up the broccoli or spinach into small pieces and put in a covered dish in the microwave with a drop of water. If you haven't got a microwave, put the broccoli in a small saucepan with enough boiling water to cover it and simmer for a couple of minutes. (If you're using spinach, it can go straight in with the rest of the ingredients.)
2. Drain the tins of tuna and sweetcorn and put them in an ovenproof dish.
3. Add the broccoli or spinach, a handful of grated cheese,

chopped tomatoes and a couple of spoonfuls of yoghurt, plus whatever seasoning you want to use and mix it all up.

4. Crush the packets of crisps and sprinkle on the top of the pie with more grated cheese and bake in a hot oven for 10–15 minutes.

ALSO TRY...

1. Instead of tinned tomatoes and yoghurt, use any, or a combination of any of the following, to make the sauce: a tin of condensed soup, crème fraiche, mayonnaise, tomato puree.
2. Include tinned broad beans and peas, or frozen mixed vegetables and peppers.
3. Instead of tuna, use a tin of salmon, or one tin each of salmon and tuna.

NOODLES

You can't go wrong with noodles, they're dirt cheap and keep for ages; kids seem to love them and it's easy to mix them up with healthier ingredients.

SERVES 4–6:
8 oz (250 g) packet of dried egg noodles
6 rashers of back bacon
Mushrooms (4–6 large approx)
Spinach (say ¼ bag)
Sesame seeds
Butter
½ pint (125 ml) vegetable or pork stock
¼ tsp nutmeg
White pepper
Parsley or chives

METHOD

1. Melt the butter in a large saucepan, snip the bacon into small pieces and fry with the sliced mushrooms and sesame seeds until everything is golden brown and the bacon is crisp.
2. Wash and tear the spinach up and add to the pan with the stock, nutmeg and pepper, stirring well.
3. Break the dried noodles up and add them to the pan, stirring again.
4. Simmer for about 5 minutes, until the noodles are just soft, serve sprinkled with parsley or chives and a small lump of butter.

MORE NOODLES

This is a good way of using up spare sausages and leftover (uncooked) mince.

SERVES 4 MEDIUM-SIZED CHILDREN

2 sausages + about 4 oz (100 g) leftover mince — or a bit of both.
3 tbsp flour, seasoned with salt and pepper
1 14 oz (400 g) tin of chopped tomatoes
Onion
Spinach (say ¼ of a bag)
½ courgette, cut into thin quarters
¼ tsp cayenne pepper
Olive oil
2–3 squares of dried noodles
Basil
Sage

METHOD

1. Roll the meat into tiny balls, about the size of a 1p coin — if you're using leftover sausages, squeeze the meat out of the sausage skins first — using the seasoned flour to coat the

meatballs. *(Mix the mince and sausage meat together if you're using both.)*
2. Fry the meatballs and courgette pieces in a couple of tablespoons of olive oil in a large saucepan or wok for a few minutes and add the chopped tomatoes. Bring to the boil and stir in the cayenne pepper with whatever other spices or herbs you want to use.
3. Tear the spinach leaves up and add to the sauce, followed by the noodles.
4. Simmer gently for a couple of minutes until the noodles are just soft. Adjust the seasoning and serve.

BACON CAKES

SERVES 4:
6 rashers of streaky bacon
2 medium-sized potatoes
1 onion, very finely chopped
2 eggs
2 tbsps self-raising flour
Salt & pepper
Oil

METHOD
1. Snip the bacon into tiny pieces, finely chop the onion, peel, wash, rinse and grate the potatoes and put everything in a mixing bowl.
2. Stir the flour and seasoning into the mixture, followed by the eggs, and beat it all together.
3. Warm the oil in a large frying pan and put spoonfuls of the mixture into the hot oil, flatten them slightly and cook for a few minutes, turning once, until the bacon cakes are crisp and brown.
4. Keep warm in the oven or under the grill (on low) and serve with baked beans.

DEVILLED KIDNEYS

Perfect with couscous when you haven't got time to cook rice; add
$\frac{1}{2}$ teaspoon of cayenne pepper or a bit more Tabasco for extra heat.

SERVES 4:
1 lb (450 – 500 g) lambs' kidneys
4 oz (100 g) streaky bacon
1 medium-sized onion
1 standard tin of chopped tomatoes
1 tsp Tabasco sauce
4 tbsp sherry
Worcester sauce
Parsley
Oregano
Butter
Oil

METHOD
1. Warm some oil and butter in a large pan; add the onion and bacon, cut up small, and fry for a few minutes until golden.
2. Rinse the kidneys in cold water, then cut into rough quarters and add them to the pan, browning quickly on all sides.
3. Stir in the chopped tomatoes with the rest of the ingredients, bring to the boil, then turn the heat down and simmer for about 10 minutes until the kidneys are cooked through and the sauce has reduced and thickened slightly.
4. Sprinkle with plenty of parsley and serve with the couscous.

ONE-STEP PASTA

Use the smallest dried pasta shapes for extra speed; the ones made especially for kids are ideal, although they tend to be more expensive. Fresh pasta requires even less cooking time – about 3 minutes – in which case, put the frankfurters in first.

SERVES 4–6:
Pasta shapes, one handful per person, roughly
Packet of 10 skinny frankfurters
Handful of frozen sweetcorn
Handful of sugar snap peas
Cherry tomatoes
Grated cheese

METHOD
1. Put the pasta into slightly salted boiling water.
2. After about 5 minutess add the sliced frankfurters and sweetcorn.
3. Put the sugar snap peas in for the last 2 minutes.
4. Strain the whole lot together when the pasta is cooked; stir in a very little olive oil or butter and serve with cherry tomatoes – or tomato ketchup if that's all you've got – and grated cheese.

INSTANT CORNED BEEF HASH

Traditionally made with leftover boiled potatoes, a very unorthodox version of corned beef hash can be made with potato purls, otherwise known as instant mash. (You may not have stooped this low before, but once you've got more than one child to transport from A to B in record time every night – or you're just too tired to care – you will, I assure you.)

If you're making this for more than four people, especially older kids and adults, you'll need to double up the quantities below.

SERVES 4:
Instant mashed potato made with milk and water according to the instructions on the packet
1 tin of corned beef
1 large onion
Oil

METHOD
1. Warm enough oil to just cover the bottom of a large frying pan, peel and thinly slice the onion; cut the corned beef into chunks.
2. Fry the corned beef and onion in the hot oil for a few minutes until brown, while you make the instant mashed potato according to the instructions on the packet.
3. Add the potato to the pan, turning it over every few seconds until it's as crisp and brown as you want it to be.
4. Serve with baked beans.

PRAWN & EGG PIE

For a deluxe version of Prawn & Egg Pie, make short crust pastry in the usual way with about ½ lb (225 g) of plain flour, then grease and line a deep-sided pie dish (or a 7″/8″ sandwich tin) and layer the ingredients, starting and finishing with grated cheese and adding beaten egg twice; once about halfway up the pie and again just before the final layer of cheese.

The quick fix Prawn & Egg Pie is equally good hot or cold and should serve four adults, but it's worth noting that you can make two pies as easily as one; all you need to do is buy an extra flan case and double up the ingredients below.

Add lemon juice, salt, black pepper, chives or basil, as you like.

TO MAKE ONE PIE:
1 readymade savoury pastry flan case (standard size 7″)
1 small packet of frozen prawns
1 tomato
1 egg
Milk
A handful of spinach
Grated cheese

METHOD
1. Wash and cut the tomato into half slices; tear or shred the spinach and rinse the prawns.
2. Beat the egg, adding a dash of milk, then mix with the rest of the ingredients, saving some of the cheese for the top of the pie.
3. Pour the filling into the flan case, spreading it out as evenly as possible, and sprinkle the remainder of the cheese.
4. Bake in the oven, Gas Mark 5 (190°C) for about 15 minutes, until the top is a light golden brown.

FISH FINGER PIE

Fish fingers (2   4 per person, depending on size of person)
Spinach
Tomatoes
Grated cheese

METHOD
1. Place fish fingers side by side in batches of 2 −4 and grill on high for 10 minutes.

2. Wash and slice the tomatoes, shred the spinach and grate the cheese.
3. Turn the fish fingers over and grill on the second side for 2 minutes; no longer.
4. Cover each batch of fish fingers with a layer of spinach and top with the slices of tomato and cheese; grill for a few more minutes and serve. *N.B. Oven chips don't take longer than half an hour, so put some on before you start if you've got another five or ten minutes to spare.*

SMOKED SALMON AND TAGLIATELLI

For extra speed use fresh tagliatelle, but be careful not to let it overcook before you return it to the pan with the smoked salmon and crème fraiche. (You could also add a few prawns at the same time if you like.)

Best served with salad (cucumber, watercress or baby leaf spinach and avocado) or green vegetables (French beans, mange tout or sugar snap peas).

SERVES 4 −6:
Tagliatelle (one generous handful per person)
3−4 slices of smoked salmon
4 tbsp crème fraiche (approx)
Baby plum or cherry tomatoes
Parsley
Balsamic vinegar

METHOD
1. Slice the smoked salmon quite thinly, halve the tomatoes and sprinkle with balsamic vinegar.
2. Prepare the salad or whichever green vegetables you want to use, according to the instructions on the packet − a couple of

minutes in the microwave should be all they need.

3. Simmer the tagliatelle in boiling water until it's *just done*, then strain through a colander.

4. Soften the crème fraiche in the still-warm pan over the lowest heat before returning the pasta to the saucepan with the smoked salmon, crème fraiche and parsley.

5. Stir well and gently warm through for a couple of minutes before serving with the tomatoes and vegetables.

FASTEST-EVER FISHCAKES

MAKES 6:

1 large tin of salmon (red or pink)
2 oz (50 g) self-raising flour
2 eggs, beaten
2 tbsp lemon juice
Parsley
Salt & pepper
Oil

METHOD

1. Drain the tin of salmon and mash the fish in a bowl with a fork. (Pick out any extra big bits of skin but leave the bones in and crush them up with the fish.)

2. Add the beaten eggs, lemon juice, seasoning and sifted flour and mix well.

3. Warm enough oil in a large frying pan to cover the bottom of the pan and drop spoonfuls of the mixture into the hot oil, pressing gently into shape with the slice and turning once. Serve with lemon wedges and salad.

THINGS ON TOAST

Just in case you need reminding, the following things are all brilliant on toast and help transform a couple of slices of bread into a makeshift meal...

1. BAKED BEANS: Spread the toast with butter and Marmite first and top the beans with grated cheese.
2. OILY FISH: Tinned sardines or mackerel in tomato sauce; both good sources of those Omega 3 fatty acids we're always hearing about. Toast the bread on one side, turn over and top with the mashed-up fish; no need for butter, but especially good with lashings of tomato ketchup.
3. TUNA AND CHEESE MELT: Tuna mixed with grated cheese; toast and serve as above.
4. CHEESE: Topped and grilled with thinly sliced tomato, or on its own with a dash of Worcester sauce, or a spoonful of sweet pickle or chutney.
5. EGGS: Scrambled or poached, with sliced ham or leftover cold sausages.
6. PATE: Chicken liver pate with mustard, or kipper pate *(see Chapter 9: Not Only, But Also)*.

ALSO TRY...
1. CHICKEN & LEEK CASSEROLE: *(see Chapter 10: Weekly Menu Planning)*.
2. OMELETTES: *(see Chapter 10: Weekly Menu Planning)*.
3. SWEET & SOUR CHICKEN: *(see Chapter 3: Make Dinner, Not Excuses)*.

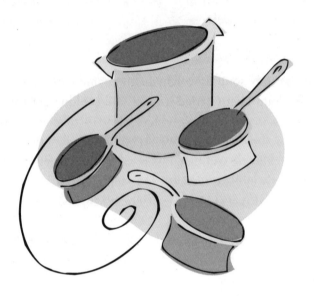

"Soup and fish explain half the
emotions of human life."

Sydney Smith

The joy of soup

There's nothing to beat good old-fashioned soup made with fresh ingredients when it comes to availability, versatility, and the art of saving money on your supermarket shopping.

About the only soup unworthy of the name is the one in the Cabbage Soup Diet (I tried it twice and couldn't get past Day Two) which is vile, and a complete waste of time and effort – everybody knows you put the weight back on the first time you eat a Malteser. Having said that, if you want to lose weight sensibly and painlessly without reducing your energy levels, you could do a lot worse than including plenty of homemade soups in your diet. All soups freeze well and can be stored in large and small amounts; for family dinners, or for taking to work and re-heating in the microwave – very handy when you want to avoid the temptations of the deli or sandwich bar.

Make soup more appealing to children by adding croutons, grated cheese and pasta shapes, or give them a bit less soup (a little goes a long way in any case) with a hot dog or toasted sandwich on the side.

You can't go far wrong with soup whatever you do, so use these recipes as a guideline and make the rest up as you go along.

Tips

To thicken soup, whisk in a couple of tablespoons of potato purls (oh how much more respectable that sounds than 'instant mash'), while the soup is still warm. Almost as outrageous as a celebrity chef using Knorr stock cubes, but there it is.

Unless otherwise specified in the recipe, add the herbs and spices mixed with the stock for even distribution.

Add a spoonful of Marmite or Vegemite to larger amounts of stock, instead of a second stock cube.

Use alternative herbs and spices if you like, but don't miss them out altogether; they do make a difference. (Buy bouquet garni ready made-up in little tea bags to save time.)

For creamed soups, pour the cream over the surface in a circular movement, straight from the carton, or create a marbled effect by zigzagging a knife or the edge of a metal spoon through the trail of cream.

ORANGE SQUASH SOUP

1 lb (500 g) carrots
1 butternut squash (any size)
1 large onion
1 small orange
1 ½ pints (750 ml) chicken or vegetable stock
1 clove of garlic
Ginger, coriander, salt & white pepper
Sunflower oil
Butter

METHOD

1. Melt the oil and butter in a large saucepan while you peel the butternut squash (removing the pips and pithy inside completely) and scrape the carrots.
2. Roughly chop the squash, carrots and onion, put them in the pan with the crushed garlic and leave to soften over a low heat for a few minutes.

3. Add the zest of half the orange to the saucepan with the ginger, coriander, salt and pepper.
4. Cut the orange into quarters and make sure the pips are removed; give each quarter a little squeeze as you add it to the pan, then pour over the chicken or vegetable stock and give it a good stir.
5. Cover with a lid, turn the heat right down and simmer gently for about 30 minutes.
6. Remove the orange quarters and throw them away.
7. Blend the soup and add salt and pepper according to taste.

SLUG & CELERY SOUP

There's an even quicker way to make this soup; just put the raw ingredients with the seasoning, milk and wine in the food processor, blend the whole lot until smooth (one minute, max), then heat it up in a large saucepan.

1 head of celery with leaves left on
1 large onion
1 clove of garlic
2 tbsp plain flour
1 pint (500 ml) chicken or vegetable stock
¼ pint (125 ml) milk
1 great big slug of white wine (say half a glass)
Celery salt or salt & white pepper
Sunflower oil
Butter

METHOD
1. Melt the butter and oil in a large saucepan.
2. Wash and chop the celery and onion and cook gently over a low heat for a few minutes with the crushed garlic.

3. Stir in the flour and cook for another minute.
4. Add the chicken or vegetable stock with the seasoning. Bring to the boil, then turn the heat right down, add the wine and milk and simmer gently for up to 30 minutes.
5. Adjust the seasoning and blend.

WATERCRESS SOUP

Another good one for speed and simplicity (not to mention a healthy dose of iron), watercress soup also doubles as a great sauce to have with any white fish or salmon.

1 or 2 bags of watercress (or a couple of large bunches) depending on size
1 onion
1 clove of garlic
2 tbsp flour
Butter
1 pint (500 ml) chicken or vegetable stock
¼ pint (125 ml) milk
Parsley
Salt & pepper
Single cream

METHOD
1. Melt the butter in a large saucepan, add the onion with the garlic and parsley and cook gently for a few minutes until the onion is soft.
2. Add the watercress, cover the pan with a lid and cook for another few minutes.
3. Stir in the flour; keep stirring for another minute, then remove the pan from the heat and add the stock and milk.

4. Bring the soup to the boil, stirring occasionally, then turn the heat down and simmer for another 5 minutes.
5. Blend the soup; add a swirl of single cream and garnish with sprigs of watercress, or sprinkle more parsley on top.

STINGING NETTLE SOUP

I've always liked the idea of making soup with nettles. There's something very appealing about a type of leaf that's plentiful, accessible, full of vitamins and minerals and – until someone decides to market stinging nettles as the latest, must-have ingredient – they're FREE!

This recipe is more or less the same as the one for watercress soup (above) and, not surprisingly, the end result also looks and tastes very similar. The difference is you need a pair of rubber gloves to make this soup; the nettles don't lose their sting until they're cooked and, as you'd expect, they also need to be washed more carefully.

Pick only the top two or three inches of the youngest, brightest green nettles you can get your hands on (ouch) and don't worry too much about the quantity; as a rough guide, the equivalent of a medium-sized bag of watercress or spinach is just fine.

Nettles
1 onion
2 cloves of garlic
1 pint (500 ml) chicken stock (2 stock cubes)
¼ pint (125 ml) milk
1 tsp nutmeg
1tbsp malt vinegar
2 heaped tbsp plain flour
2 tsp dried parsley
Butter
Salt & pepper

METHOD

1. Wearing rubber gloves, plunge the nettles into a bowl of cold water with lots of salt, and fish them out a few at a time to wash properly in another bowl of cold water, or under the tap, until you're sure they're clean. (Remove any big, tough stalks if there are any, otherwise the leaves can stay attached to the stems.)
2. Warm some butter in a large saucepan while you peel and chop the onion and crush the garlic, then put them in the pan and cook gently for a few minutes until the onion has softened.
3. Squeeze excess water from the nettles – still wearing the rubber gloves – and add them to the pan with a spoonful of vinegar. Cover the pan with a lid and simmer gently for about 5 minutes before adding the chicken stock, milk and nutmeg.
4. Stir well and bring the soup to the boil while you mash 2 heaped tablespoons of plain flour, 1 tablespoon of butter and 2 teaspoons of dried parsley in a cup or bowl, until smooth.
5. As soon as the nettle soup has started to boil, turn the heat right down and add the parsley butter and flour mixture, stir until dissolved, then leave to simmer gently for about 5 minutes.
6. Blend the soup and garnish each serving with a fresh sprig of nettle. (Only joking.)

SWEET POTATO SOUP

2 sweet potatoes
2–3 carrots
1 onion
3-4 rashers of bacon (streaky or back)
1 tbsp flour
2 pints (1 litre) chicken or vegetable stock (2 stock cubes)
Salt & pepper
1 tbsp butter

METHOD

1. Wash and chop the vegetables and make the stock.
2. Melt the butter in a large pan and pop the bacon in for a couple of minutes on its own, then add the vegetables and fry for a further five minutes.
3. Add the flour and cook for a minute.
4. Stir in the stock, bring to the boil, cover with a lid and simmer for about 30 minutes, until all the vegetables are soft.
5. Allow to cool for a few minutes and blend.

LENTIL & VEGETABLE SOUP

There's no end to what you can do with lentils and vegetables; use red or yellow lentils if you want to avoid soaking the lentils in advance, otherwise, brown and green lentils or chick peas will do the job.

8 oz (approx 200 g) red lentils
2 small potatoes
½ small swede
2–3 carrots
2 –3 sticks of celery
1 smallish parsnip
1 onion
2 cloves of garlic
2 pints (1 litre) vegetable stock (2 stock cubes)
Salt & pepper
Oil
Parsley

OPTIONAL:

1 level tsp curry powder

METHOD

1. Warm the oil in a very large saucepan and gently fry the onion and garlic until the onion is soft.
2. Add the lentils and cook for one minute.
3. Add the rest of the vegetables and seasoning and cook on a low heat for another 5 minutes or so.
4. Add the stock, bring to the boil, then reduce the heat and simmer for 20 –30 minutes until the vegetables are soft.
5. Blend, adjust the seasoning and serve garnished with parsley.

SPICY BEAN SOUP

Beans are good for your heart, the more you eat the more you realise how easy it is to make something nourishing with them.

High in fibre, low in fat and cheaper than chips; use fresh beans if you like (they're even cheaper), but tinned ones are normally just as good. You'll find all of the beans listed here beside the baked beans in the supermarket.

This soup isn't blended at the end, so slice or dice the vegetables finely, the way you want them to look in the finished soup.

Any 2 (different) tins of beans from the following list: borlotti beans, butter beans, broad beans, canellini beans, kidney beans, chick peas

2 courgettes

2 carrots

2 sticks of celery

1 onion

4 rashers of back bacon (rind and fat removed)

2 cloves of garlic
2 pints (1 litre) beef, lamb or pork stock
2 bay leaves
1 level tsp curry powder or cumin
Worcester sauce
½ tsp mixed spice
2–3 tbsp potato purls
Oil

METHOD
1. Heat the oil in a very large pan and prepare the vegetables, then snip the bacon into small pieces and fry until crisp and golden.
2. Add the finely chopped celery, carrots, courgettes, onion and garlic and fry for another 10 minutes until everything looks ready.
3. Add the stock with the spices and bay leaves mixed in and simmer for 15–20 minutes.
4. Drain the tins of beans, add them to the soup and simmer for another 5 minutes.
5. To finish: sprinkle the potato purls into the soup, whisking with a small hand whisk or a fork until dissolved.

TOMATO & RED LENTIL SOUP

This can be thinned down and used as the sauce for a pasta bake (*see Salmon & Tomato Bake, Chapter 10: Weekly Menu Planning*).

It goes without saying that you can always use fresh ingredients instead of tinned if you want to, so if you're using fresh tomatoes for this, put them in a pan of very hot water for a minute, then fish them out with a slotted spoon; the skin should peel away easily and they're ready to use.

2 –3 tins of chopped or plum tomatoes (or 2 lbs (1 kg) of fresh)
8 oz (200 g) red lentils
4 rashers of streaky bacon
2 onions
2 ½ pints (1.25 litres) chicken stock (2 stock cubes)
1 tsp brown sugar
Basil
Salt & pepper
Butter
Olive oil

METHOD

1. Peel and roughly chop the onion, snip the bacon into pieces and wash the lentils thoroughly in a sieve or colander.
2. Melt a little butter with some olive oil in a large saucepan and fry the onion and bacon for a few minutes until golden.
3. Add the lentils to the pan, followed by the tomatoes, stock and seasoning and stir well.
4. Bring to the boil and simmer gently for about 30 minutes.
5. Blend the soup; adjust the seasoning and, if necessary, thin it down with a little more stock, milk, or tomato juice, according to taste and requirements.

MINESTRONE

Use whichever beans you like; borlotti, canellini, kidney beans, chick peas or mixed beans.

4 oz (100 g) or ½ cup of small pasta shapes, such as farfallini
4–6 rashers of streaky bacon
1 onion
1 small green and 1 red pepper

2 courgettes

2 carrots

2 celery sticks

1 tin of chopped tomatoes

1 tin of beans

2 cloves of garlic

2 ½ pints (1.25 litres) chicken stock (2 stock cubes)

Oregano or Italian herbs

Basil

1 tsp soft brown sugar

Pepper

Olive oil

Crouton

Parmesan/grated cheese

METHOD

1. Warm a little oil in a very large saucepan and fry the bacon and onion until crisp and golden while you prepare the rest of the vegetables. (Don't add anything else to the pan too soon or you'll never get the bacon crisp.)
2. Add the celery, courgettes, carrots, peppers and garlic, followed by the chopped tomatoes and the chicken stock mixed with the herbs and sugar.
3. Stir well, bring to the boil and simmer gently for about 10 minutes.
4. Add the pasta and the tinned beans and simmer for another 15–20 minutes, until the vegetables and pasta are just soft.
5. Season to taste (add a little tomato puree if you like) and serve with croutons and parmesan, or any other grated cheese.

SMOKED MACKEREL CHOWDER

Don't worry too much about the size and weight of the fish, or the number of fillets in the packet; the chowder will turn out okay however much fish you use.

1 packet of smoked mackerel fillets
1 ½ pints (750 ml) milk (whole or semi-skimmed)
Potatoes (say 4 medium-sized or 6 small)
2 leeks
1 onion
2 serving spoons frozen sweetcorn
¼ pint (125 ml) single cream
1 tbsp flour
Dried parsley, roughly 2 tsp – or more, according to taste
Butter
Oil

METHOD
1. Peel and chop the potatoes into small chunks; wash and finely chop the onion and leeks.
2. Melt butter and oil in a large saucepan and gently brown the potatoes for a few minutes. Add the onion and leeks and fry for a few more minutes until the onion has softened, then stir in the flour and cook for another minute.
3. Add the frozen sweetcorn, pour in the milk with the cream and bring to the boil while you remove the skin from the mackerel and flake the fish, making sure there aren't any bones.
4. Turn the heat right down and add the mackerel to the pan with the parsley, stir well and leave to simmer for about 20 minutes, or until the potatoes are just soft.

5. If you want to thicken the chowder at the end, add a little corn flour or 1 tbsp plain flour to another 2 tbsp cream. For a thinner consistency, just add more milk.

MEAT SOUPS

Soups in which meat is the main ingredient naturally take longer to cook, but the preparation is still straightforward – and once the soup's cooking you can go off and do something else.

BORSHT

I hated beetroot as a child, and even though it's never going to be one of my favourite vegetables (I still can't stand it pickled in vinegar), I do like borsht. It probably helps that I put less beetroot and more beef in mine than in some of the other recipes I've seen, so if you also think you hate beetroot, give borsht a try; you might be pleasantly surprised.

About 2 lb (1 kg) stewing or braising steak
2 fresh, raw beetroots
½ small white cabbage
1 carrot
1–2 sticks of celery
1 onion studded with a few cloves
Bouquet garni
1 14 oz (410 g) can of chopped tomatoes
Tomato puree
2 bay leaves
2 tsp brown sugar
1 small carton sour cream

METHOD

1. Trim any fat off the meat and cut into small, even pieces, then put in a large saucepan with 2 pints (1 litre) of fresh, cold water.
2. Peel the onion, leaving it whole, and stick a few cloves into it.
3. Wash the carrot and celery sticks; leave them whole or cut them in half so they're easier to fish out of the pan later on.
4. Put the onion, carrot, celery and bouquet garni into the pan with the meat; turn the heat up high and bring to the boil.
5. When the water is boiling, turn the heat right down, skin the scum off the top with a slotted spoon, cover with a lid again and leave the soup to simmer very gently for about 30 minutes.
6. Meanwhile, peel and cut the beetroot into matchstick-sized pieces and finely shred the cabbage.
7. When the meat is *almost* tender, get rid of the carrots, onion, celery and bouquet garni, and use a cup or ladle to remove about ¼ of the liquid.
8. Add the beetroot, cabbage and the rest of the ingredients – tinned tomatoes, tomato puree, sugar and bay leaves and simmer very gently for about 1 hour, until the beef is very tender.
9. When you think the soup is ready, pick the bay leaves out, and if you want the soup to be a bit less liquid, thicken it with a tablespoon of butter mixed with 1 tbsp plain flour.
10. Add sour cream to the Borsht to finish, and serve with soda bread.

CHICKEN SOUP

Use the chicken carcass to make the stock for chicken soup; it's a lot less hassle than you might think. It doesn't matter whether you use the whole chicken or just the remains, but ideally you should have at least one-third of the meat left for the soup.

This soup is half blended, so cut the vegetables for the finished soup into smaller pieces than you would for the stock.

FOR THE STOCK:
Chicken carcass
3 –4 pints (2 litres) fresh, cold water
2 carrots
2 sticks of celery
1 onion
2 bay leaves
4 black peppercorns

FOR THE SOUP:
1 small/medium organic, free-range chicken (cooked)
2+ pints (1.2 litres) fresh chicken stock
3 medium-sized potatoes
2 –3 carrots
2 –3 sticks of celery
1 onion
1 bouquet garni
Oil/butter

OPTIONAL:
Thyme or tarragon
Salt & pepper
¼ pint (125 ml) single cream

METHOD
TO MAKE THE STOCK:
1. Remove the skin and as much meat as you can from the cooked chicken; discard the skin and set the meat aside.
2. Put the chicken carcass in a very large pot with the bay leaves, peppercorns, onion, carrots and celery; washed and roughly chopped, and cover with fresh, cold water.
3. Bring to the boil then turn the heat right down and simmer

gently for up to 4 hours – or longer if you have time, but ideally, no less than 2 hours.

4. When you're ready, remove the chicken carcass, vegetables and bay leaves and give the stock a good stir with a slotted spoon to make sure it's clear. *N.B. If you think you've got a lot more stock than you want for the quantity of soup you're making, take out what you don't need now and keep it in the fridge for a couple of days, or freeze it for up to 3 months.*

To make the soup:

1. Cut the potatoes, carrots, celery and onion into small pieces and fry them in oil or butter (or a bit of both) for a few minutes, in a very large saucepan.

2. Add the stock with the herbs and the bouquet garni *(see notes, page 120)*, bring to the boil and simmer gently for about 30 minutes, until the vegetables are tender but not mushy.

3. Remove the bouquet garni and blend half of the soup. Mix the remainder of the soup with the blended half and add the chicken, cut into small pieces. Warm the soup thoroughly, adding the cream at the end. *N.B. If you're making the soup for later, rather than eating it straightaway, allow the soup to cool before adding the chicken pieces.*

SCOTCH BROTH

The first and, until recently, the last time I made Scotch Broth was at school, which, thinking about it now, must be an indication of two things; one, how times have changed, and two, how simple this must be if a thirteen-year-old could make it. (It was perfectly edible as well; we ate what I made at home.)

I can't for the life of me think why I haven't made it before now, not least because it's great to be able to buy cheaper cuts of meat, knowing all it takes is a little time and gentle cooking to make it as tender and delicious as the more expensive ones.

I used 1 ½ lb (725 g) of neck fillet (if you have a butcher, ask for scrag end of lamb) or if you prefer, use a similar amount of beef stewing steak.

1 –2 lb (500 g–1 kg) meat
2–3 carrots
2 leeks
½ small Swede or 2–3 turnips, depending on size
2 onions
5 –6 tbsp pearl barley
2 lamb or beef stock cubes
Parsley
Salt & pepper

METHOD

1. Cut up the meat with kitchen scissors; put the pieces in a large saucepan with enough water to cover – about 2 ½ pints (1.5 litres) – and simmer with a lid on for 1 ½ hours. (Skim the fat off the surface once or twice.)
2. 10–15 minutes before the end of cooking time, wash, peel and dice the vegetables.
3. Put the barley into a small saucepan with just enough cold water to cover; boil for a few minutes before straining through a sieve and rinsing under the cold tap. (You don't have to blanch the barley this way but it helps to prevent a scum forming on the finished soup.)
4. Add the barley, vegetables, parsley and stock cubes to the pan with the meat and simmer very gently for about 30 minutes until the vegetables and barley are just soft.
5. Serve the broth, adding as much of the liquid broth from the pan as you want.

CHILLED SOUPS

COOL CUCUMBER SOUP

The look of this soup is greatly improved by a few drops of green food colouring, but if you want to keep it as natural as possible (or you don't happen to have green food colouring) it won't matter too much if you leave it out.

2 large cucumbers
1 small onion
1 pint (500 ml) warm milk
½ pint (250 ml) chicken stock (1 stock cube)
1 tbsp plain flour
½ tsp nutmeg
Salt & pepper
Butter
1 small carton of single cream
Mint

METHOD
1. Peel and halve the cucumbers, cut out the seedy bit in the middle and chop the cucumbers into chunks; peel and chop the onion.
2. Melt some butter in a large saucepan, fry the cucumber and onion for a few minutes before adding the flour and cooking for another minute, stirring all the time.
3. Meanwhile, warm the milk in another saucepan and make ½ pint (250 ml) of stock with 1 stock cube in a measuring jug, adding the nutmeg and seasoning to the hot stock.
4. Remove the pan with the vegetables from the heat and gradually pour on the stock and warm milk, stirring continuously.

5. Bring the soup to the boil, still stirring, then turn the heat right down and simmer gently for about 20 minutes.
6. Allow the soup to cool for a few minutes then puree in a blender or food processor; adjust the seasoning and add a few drops of green food colouring, if you're using it.
7. Chill the soup in the fridge for at least 2 hours; serve with a swirl of single cream and a sprinkling of mint.

HOT OR COLD LEEK & POTATO SOUP

This is basically a recipe for Vichyssoise, a classic cold soup, but it's also very good hot ... so over to you.

1 lb (450 g) leeks
1 lb (450 g) potatoes
1 medium onion
1 ½ pints (750 ml) chicken stock
1 clove of garlic
Chives
Butter
Oil
1 small carton single cream
Salt & pepper

METHOD
1. Peel the potatoes, rinse well and cut into small chunks; also top and tail and slice the leeks, and chop the onion.
2. Warm butter and oil in a large saucepan, add crushed garlic and the vegetables, then cover the pan with a lid and cook gently for a few minutes.
3. Pour on the stock, season with salt and pepper and bring to the boil, then turn the heat down and simmer gently for

20–30 minutes until the vegetables are just soft.

4. Allow to cool for a few minutes, then puree the soup, blending thoroughly until the soup is very smooth. Adjust the seasoning, then either chill the soup in the fridge for a couple of hours, or re-heat when ready to use. Hot or cold, finish the soup with single cream and a sprinkling of chives.

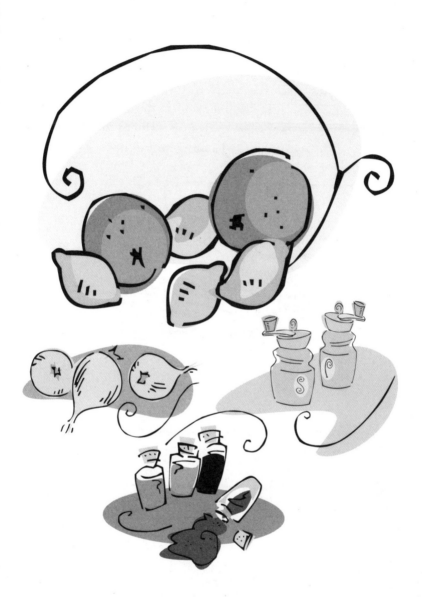

"Part of the secret of success in life is
to eat what you like and let the food
fight it out inside."

Mark Twain

Join the pudding club

Pudding as an everyday thing fell out of fashion years ago, which is hardly surprising when we're obsessed with healthy eating, more women than ever are out at work and you can already buy everything from profiteroles to pavlova in the supermarket.

But it can't be right that the nation who gave the world spotted dick and treacle tart (not to mention apple pie, which is English whatever they think in America) should give up homemade puddings altogether and settle for a gloomy future of frozen lemon meringue pie, so if you think you haven't got time for puddings, think again. Plenty of desserts take only a minimal amount of time and effort, and there's nothing like the promise of something sweet for getting kids to dutifully eat more of the things you really want them to have first.

Having said that, desserts and puddings, or whatever you want to call them, aren't necessarily an unhealthy option either, especially when they contain a lot of fruit, and as a truly satisfying comfort food they do a lot less damage to your diet than a family-sized bar of chocolate or a bag of doughnuts.

Try and make puddings a part of your life; even once a week is better than never. Your family and friends will love you for it.

Tips

Pour evaporated milk (Carnation) over fresh and tinned fruit puddings as a cheap and easy alternative to cream or custard.

Buy golden syrup and maple syrup in plastic bottles for easy squeezing.

Cool jelly quickly by adding slightly less cold water to the melted jelly and popping 2 or 3 ice cubes in.

Make sour cream by adding 1 tablespoon of lemon juice to a small carton (5 floz/150 ml) of single cream.

Make chocolate custard simply by mixing 1 oz (25 g) of chocolate into warm custard, readymade or instant; or melt the chocolate in the microwave first and stir it in.

PASTRY

A basic short crust pastry is all you'll ever need for most pies and flans; add 1 level tablespoon of caster or icing sugar to make it slightly sweeter – and replace half the quantity of fat with lard, which gives the pastry more of a melt-in-the-mouth quality, if you want to. The quantities given below make enough pastry to line a shallow, loose-bottomed 8″ (15cm) flan tin.

SHORT CRUST PASTRY:

6 oz (150 g) plain flour

3 oz (75 g) butter or margarine (or 1 ½ oz [33 g] each of butter and lard)

1 heaped tbsp caster sugar (or icing sugar)

4 tbsp cold water (approx)

METHOD

1. Sift the flour into a very large mixing bowl and rub in the butter or margarine in small pieces until the mixture resembles fine breadcrumbs.
2. Stir in the sugar, make a well in the centre, then add the water or milk, gradually incorporating the flour by pinching the mixture together with the fingers of one hand. Knead the pastry inside the bowl for a minute to make a firm, smooth dough.
3. Wrap the dough in foil or a double layer of clingfilm and chill in the fridge for half an hour before turning the dough onto a

floured surface and rolling it out to fit the lightly greased flan tin, or pie dish.

4. Prick the pastry with a fork several times before adding the filling. If the pastry case is to be baked 'blind' – i.e. on its own so the filling can be added when the pastry is cold – cover with a circle of greaseproof paper then weigh the paper down with a handful of dried beans, lentils or rice.

5. Bake in the oven, Gas Mark 4 (180°C) for 10–15 minutes. (Remove dried beans and greaseproof paper and return to the oven for a further 5 minutes to crisp the pastry.)

If you also have an irrational fear of recipes containing gelatine, these are the cheesecakes for you...

CHERRY CHEESECAKE

If you can't find the exact quantities of cherries and cream cheese mentioned here, get the nearest sizes up, and if the cherries aren't pitted, remove the stones yourself by making a little cut down one side of the fruit with a sharp knife and gently squeezing the stone out.

An even easier option is to buy a tin of cherry pie filling, mix half with the beaten cream cheese and spread the remainder over the top of the cheesecake, thinning it with a little fruit juice first, if need be.

SERVES 4–6:
FOR THE BISCUIT BASE:
8 large digestive biscuits, crushed by hand
2 oz (50 g) butter

FOR THE CHEESECAKE:
15 oz (425 g) tin of black cherries in heavy syrup

1 rounded tbsp cornflour

1 heaped tbsp sugar (white or soft brown)

2 tbsp Amaretto (or similar liqueur)

½ lb (300 g) tub of soft cream cheese

METHOD

1. Lightly grease a round, loose-bottomed cake tin, approx 6″/7″ (12 cm)
2. Make the biscuit base by melting the butter in a saucepan and adding the crushed digestives. (You can make biscuit crumbs in a food processor, but it only takes a minute to crush the biscuits up in a large bowl using your thumbs or a china mug.)
3. Press the biscuit mixture into the prepared tin and chill in the fridge for about 30 minutes.
4. Separate the cherries from the syrup and cut the cherries in half.
5. Pour the syrup into a saucepan with the liqueur, add the cornflour and stir quickly and constantly over a medium heat for a few minutes until the syrup becomes thick and smooth, like a gel.
6. Remove the pan from the heat, add the cherries and mix together.
7. To make the filling, beat the cream cheese in a bowl until smooth (only takes a few seconds with a wooden spoon), then add half the cherries and blend with the beaten cream cheese.
8. Spread the filling over the chilled biscuit base and top with the remainder of the cherries.
9. Chill for at least an hour and serve with single cream.

LEMON CHEESECAKE

This cheesecake works well with a pastry or a biscuit base (use a readymade sweet pastry flan case if you don't have time to make one) and, needless to say, you can use any flavour jelly with a mixture of whatever tinned and fresh fruit you like.

SERVES 4–6:
1 lemon jelly
½ lb (300 g) tub of soft cream cheese
2 tbsp crème fraiche
8 large digestive biscuits
2 oz (50 g) butter

TO DECORATE:
Kiwi fruit
Strawberries

METHOD
1. Put the jelly in a measuring jug with ½ pint (250 ml) of boiling water and stir for a few minutes until dissolved. *Don't top up with cold water in the usual way;* add 2 or 3 ice cubes to cool the jelly down quickly, then leave it to stand for 20–30 minutes. (It doesn't matter if you don't have any ice; just leave the jelly to stand in a cool place for the same amount of time.)
2. Put the cream cheese in a large mixing bowl with the cool jelly and crème fraiche and beat it all together with an electric hand whisk for half a minute until smooth.
3. Spread the filling evenly over the base and leave to set in the fridge for at least an hour.
4. Decorate the top of the cheesecake with thin slices of strawberry, kiwi fruit and tinned peaches – or whatever else you fancy.

CHESHIRE TART

Not a footballer's wife, Cheshire Tart is actually a baked cheesecake; rich, cheap, easy to make...and still not a gelatine leaf in sight.

SERVES 4–6:

FOR THE BASE:

8 large digestive biscuits

4 ginger biscuits

¹⁄₂ tsp ginger

3 oz (75 g) butter

1 tbsp golden syrup

FOR THE FILLING:

¹⁄₂ lb (300 g) tub of soft cream cheese

4 oz (100 g) Cheshire Cheese, finely grated

3 eggs, separated

2 tbsp natural yoghurt or crème fraiche

2 tsp sugar

2 tbsp lemon juice

METHOD

1. Make the biscuit base in the usual way; crushing the biscuits by hand, then mixing thoroughly with the melted butter and golden syrup.

2. Lightly grease and base-line a loose-bottomed 6″/7″ (12 cm) cake tin and press the biscuit mixture into the tin.

3. Separate the eggs into two large mixing bowls and add the grated Cheshire cheese, cream cheese, yoghurt or crème fraiche, sugar and lemon juice to the bowl with the egg yolks.

4. First whisk the egg whites (with an electric hand whisk) until they stand up in peaks and all the bubbles have disappeared; then whisk together the ingredients in the second bowl.

5. Gently fold the egg whites into the cheese mixture until the ingredients are combined, then pour the mixture onto the biscuit base and bake in a cool oven, Gas Mark 2 (150°C) for 45 minutes–1 hour, until the top is firm and set and slightly golden.

6. Allow the cheesecake to cool in the tin for about an hour, then run a sharp knife around the edge and carefully lift it out.
7. Dust the top of the cheesecake with icing sugar and serve with fresh fruit and single cream.

BAKED APPLES

You could say baked apples are a quick-fix pudding; they take no more than five minutes to prepare and you can put them in the oven as you're taking the main course out, so they'll be ready to eat straight after dinner. (They also make a nice change for a weekend breakfast with yoghurt and honey or crème fraiche.)

If you haven't got an apple corer, remove the centre of the apples by putting them on a hard, flat surface and pushing a sharp knife through each one four times in a square shape around the stalk, making sure you go right to the bottom every time; then turn the apple over and repeat the process from the other end. Now use your thumb to push the core out.

(Stick two or three cloves into the apple and remove after cooking, for extra flavour.)

1 large Bramley cooking apple per person with:
    sultanas or mixed fruit with mixed spice and brown sugar or
    chopped dried apricots with golden syrup and cinnamon or
    dried cranberries and caster sugar.

METHOD
1. Wash the apples, remove the cores and score a line all the way around each apple, halfway down and about ½ inch (1 cm) deep.
2. Mix the fruit with the sugar and spices in a small bowl.
3. Place the apples in an ovenproof dish and stuff with as much of the fruit as you can get in the middle of each apple,

scattering whatever's left over around the base.

4. Cover loosely with foil and bake in a moderate oven, Gas Mark 4 (180°C) for about 40 minutes, or until the apples are just soft. Remove the cloves and serve with cream, crème fraiche, evaporated milk or custard.

RHUBARB CRUMBLE

To me, crumbles are the perfect alternative to pies, because you get the same amount of satisfaction and enjoyment from making and eating them for less than half the effort – brilliant.

Instead of rhubarb use a similar quantity of apples, or apples and blackberries, or a combination of apples and tinned fruit – cherries, mixed summer fruits or apricots, for example – and add mixed spice, cinnamon or ground cloves, according to taste. (But unlike some people whose secret is safe with me, I haven't got the cheek to make an apple crumble with tinned apples and put cloves in it...)

As for the crumble mixture; add a couple of tablespoons of porridge oats or crunched-up cornflakes, or a smaller spoonful of ground almonds or desiccated coconut if you want to jazz it up a bit.

SERVES 4–6:
2 lb (1 kg) rhubarb
8 heaped tbsp plain flour
4 oz (100 g) butter
Sugar: Demerara, soft brown, or white
1 rounded tsp ginger
Golden syrup

METHOD
1. Top and tail the rhubarb, wash and cut into inch-long (2 cm) pieces.
2. Put the rhubarb in a saucepan with the ginger, a couple of tablespoons of sugar, a very little cold water and a modest dollop of golden syrup.
3. Simmer gently over a very low heat until the rhubarb is soft and the liquid syrupy (around 20 minutes), then transfer to a deep-sided ovenproof dish.
4. Make the crumble topping by sifting the flour into a large bowl, then adding the butter in small pieces and rubbing in until the mixture resembles fine breadcrumbs.
5. Stir another couple of tablespoons of sugar into the crumble mixture; loosely cover the fruit with the crumble without pressing it down too hard, and bake in the oven, Gas Mark 5 (190°C) for about 20 minutes, until the topping is slightly golden.

POOR MAN'S APPLE PIE

1 ½ lb (750 g) English eating apples
Cornflakes
Brown sugar
Butter

SERVES 4–6:
METHOD
1. Peel, core and thinly slice the apples and put a layer of fruit across the bottom of a medium-sized ovenproof dish.
2. Add a layer of cornflakes, then sprinkle over 1 dessert spoonful of sugar and dot with a few small pieces of butter.
3. Add another layer of apple followed by the same amount of sugar and butter, building up the layers as described above

until you run out of fruit.

4. Bake in a moderate oven, Gas Mark 4 (180°C) for about 20 minutes, until the apple is soft.

JIMMY YOUNG TRIFLE

Jimmy Young had a hugely popular 'Listener's Recipe' spot on his BBC radio show for more years than most of us can remember, which is where my mum got the idea for this banana and orange trifle (originally supplied by Mrs Audrey Hurst from Bramley in Surrey), known for ever afterwards in our house as Jimmy Young Trifle.

It's especially good if you like the idea of trifle but can't stand cold custard.

SERVES 4–6:
1 small tin of mandarin segments
2 small bananas
1 orange jelly
½ pint (250 ml) boiling water
1 swiss roll or an angel cake
¼ pint (125 ml) evaporated milk

METHOD
1. Put the jelly in a measuring jug with ½ pint (250 ml) of boiling water, stir until dissolved then add the juice from the mandarin segments, and 2 or 3 ice cubes if you have them, to make the jelly up to just ¾ pint (375 ml). Allow to cool for about 10 minutes while you arrange the pieces of cake (or a packet of trifle sponges) in a large glass bowl with the mandarin segments and chopped bananas.
2. Pour ½ pint (250 ml) of the cool jelly over the sponge and fruit and refrigerate.

3. Leave the remaining ¼ pint (125 ml) of jelly to cool completely – say another 5 minutes – then add ¼ (125 ml) pint of evaporated milk to the jug and whisk by hand for a couple of minutes until frothy. (The level of liquid in the jug should now be near the ¾ pint (375 ml) mark.)

4. Carefully pour the milk jelly over the trifle and return to the fridge to set for a couple of hours. Serve the trifle as it is, or finish it off with whipped cream and decorate with fruit or grated chocolate.

BREAD & BUTTER PUDDING

SERVES 4–6:
10 slices of medium or thinly sliced white bread, crusts removed
3 eggs
3 egg yolks
Vanilla essence, few drops
3–4 heaped tbsp caster sugar
½ pint (250 ml) milk
Small carton of single cream
½ mug of sultanas
Icing sugar

METHOD

1. Remove crusts, lightly butter the bread on both sides, then cut the slices in half diagonally and arrange them in an ovenproof dish (preferably Pyrex).

2. Wash and dry the sultanas and sprinkle over the bread.

3. Warm the milk and single cream together in a saucepan while you beat the eggs, egg yolks and vanilla essence in a bowl, then whisk in the warm milk and cream.

4. Pour the egg and milk mixture over the bread and sultanas and

gently press down with a fork or a potato masher before leaving the pudding to soak for up to half an hour (no less than 10 minutes).

5. Cover the dish with foil and place in a large roasting tin half-filled with hot water (make sure there's at least 1 inch (2 cm) between the level of water and the top of the dish) and bake in the oven, Gas Mark 4 (180°C) for about 45 minutes.

6. Remove the foil and allow the bread & butter pudding to cool for about 10 minutes before dusting with icing sugar. Serve with thick cream.

RASPBERRY ICE-CREAM

This is no match for Ben & Jerry's, but it's still pretty good – especially compared with the cheapest toxic supermarket own-brand stuff – and can be made (almost) as easily without a proper ice-cream making machine.

Make it around the same time as the bread & butter pudding (see above) and you'll be able to use up the leftover egg whites. (The really lazy way is to crush up four or five meringue nests to use instead of egg whites.)

SERVES 4–6:
14 oz (425 g) carton of ready-made custard
½ lb (225 g) of fresh raspberries
½ a large (500 g) carton of natural yoghurt
1 small carton of double cream (approx 125 ml)
3 egg whites (or 4–5 meringue nests)

METHOD
1. Briefly blend the raspberries to a rough puree or squash them up a bit with a spoon.

2. Whip the double cream in a large mixing bowl for a minute until it starts to thicken, but is still quite loose and sloppy, then stir in the custard and raspberries, mixing well to spread the fruit around and add colour.

3. Add the crushed meringue nests, or whisk the egg whites in a separate bowl and fold them into the mixture.

4. Transfer the ice-cream into the largest-size freezer bag (or a 2 litre lunch box) and put it in the freezer for about 45 minutes.

5. After 45 minutes, take the ice-cream out (stand the freezer bag in a bowl to give it some support) then stir the ice-cream with a metal spoon, or whisk it for a few seconds on the lowest setting before returning to the freezer.

6. After an hour, take the ice-cream out again and repeat STEP 5; breaking the ice-cream up to prevent ice crystals forming.

7. Repeat this process three or four times – which is why it's better to start making the ice-cream in the morning – then leave the ice-cream in the freezer, taking it out to soften up a bit about half an hour before serving.

CHOCOLATE MOUSSE

Use caster or granulated sugar if you haven't got icing sugar, and if you want a cream instead of a lighter mousse, add a couple of tablespoons of double cream or crème fraiche after the egg whites.

SERVES 6:
8 oz (225 g) plain chocolate
4 eggs
1 tsp coffee dissolved in 4 tbsp boiling water
1 tbsp sherry or brandy
1 level tbsp icing sugar

METHOD

1. Dissolve the coffee in the boiling water.
2. Break the chocolate into pieces and melt in a bowl over a saucepan of boiling water with the coffee and sherry, stirring occasionally, while you separate the eggs.
3. Once the chocolate mixture is completely smooth, remove from the heat and leave to cool for a minute before you beat the egg yolks into the mixture.
4. Whisk the egg whites in a separate bowl until stiff; add the icing sugar, then whisk for another minute until stiff enough to stand up in peaks.
5. Fold the beaten egg whites into the chocolate mixture and spoon into six glass bowls or ramekins.
6. Chill for at least 3 hours and serve with thick cream and a dusting of icing sugar and cocoa powder.

TREACLE TART

Nowadays, treacle tarts tend to be made with golden syrup; originally they were made with black treacle, so this is a modern compromise between the two. Eaten cold on its own, treacle tart is delicious; warm with extra thick cream it's to die for.

SERVES 4–6:
Short crust pastry
5 oz (125 g) fresh white breadcrumbs
6 tbsp golden syrup
2 tbsp black treacle
1 oz (25 g) butter
1 lemon, juice and rind
2 fl oz (60 ml) milk

METHOD

1. Make short crust pastry with 6 oz (150 g) plain flour (*see page 142*), then roll the pastry out to fit a lightly greased 8″ (15 cm) loose-bottomed flan tin, saving the trimmings to re-roll and cut into 8 thin strips for the top of the tart.

2. Put the syrup, treacle, butter and lemon juice in a saucepan over a low heat for a few minutes to melt the butter and dissolve the syrup and treacle.

3. Fill the pastry case to the top with the breadcrumbs, then carefully pour on the warm liquid, starting from the outside and working slowly around to the middle of the tart so all the breadcrumbs are covered.

4. Roll out the remainder of the pastry, cut out 8 thin strips, then dunk them in a small bowl of milk and make a criss-cross pattern across the top of the tart, gently pressing the ends of each strip into the edge of the pastry crust. (Mix the milk with an egg yolk for a deeper glaze.)

5. Bake in the oven, Gas Mark 4 (180°C) for 20–25 minutes until the filling is just set and the pastry a light golden brown.

TIRAMISU

This shortcut version (what else?) of tiramisu can be made in one large bowl but looks prettier piled into individual glass dessert dishes; the quantities given here will make at least six, depending on the size of your glasses. Tiramisu also freezes well and keeps for a at least two days in the fridge, meaning you can make it well in advance of a lunch or dinner party.

(Incidentally, this is one quick fix I don't feel the slightest bit guilty about since Gordon Ramsay and Jamie Oliver both have recipes for tiramisu made with sponge fingers in their books!)

SERVES APPROX 6:

1 packet (200 g) of sugar-coated sponge fingers

2 x 9 oz (250 g) tubs of mascarpone

1 medium-sized carton (500g) of custard

2 tbsp caster sugar

4 oz (100 g) bar of plain chocolate, grated

1 tbsp instant coffee dissolved in ½ pint (250 ml) of boiling water

4 tbsp Tia Mia, brandy or sherry

METHOD

1. Make ½ pint (250 ml) of coffee with 1 level tablespoon of instant coffee; add the liqueur and sugar and stir.
2. Beat the cheese in a large mixing bowl with a wooden spoon until soft, then add the custard and blend thoroughly.
3. Dip the biscuits into the coffee, put them into the glasses (3 or 4 biscuits per layer, per glass), then sprinkle a layer of grated chocolate and top with a couple of spoonfuls of the mascarpone mixture.
4. Repeat STEP 3, saving a little of the grated chocolate to sprinkle on the top of each dessert at the end.

FRUIT FOOL

The cheat's way of making a fruit fool is not to fiddle around soaking and stewing fresh fruit ... open a tin! Instead of prunes, use the same-sized tin of gooseberries, strawberries or rhubarb and add a couple of tablespoons of sherry, a few drops of vanilla extract, or the finely grated rind of half an orange to the fruit, for variation.

SERVES 4–6:

14 oz (approx 410 g) tin of prunes in natural juice or syrup
1 small (425 g) carton of custard
1 small carton (5 fl oz/ 150 ml) of double cream

METHOD

1. Tip the tinned fruit into a bowl; slit the prunes down one side with a sharp knife and pick the stones out.
2. Puree the prunes in a blender or food processor with about half the juice or syrup from the tin, then return to the bowl and stir in the carton of custard.
3. Whip the double cream in another bowl until it's firm enough to hold its shape and stand up in stiff peaks, then fold into the prunes and custard, blending thoroughly.
4. Chill in the fridge for at least two hours.

SPOTTED DICK

And here it is, hiding away at the end of the chapter for fear of being laughed at. It wouldn't be right to call this the *piéce de resistance* when Spotted Dick is English to the core – but will somebody please come up with another name for this sweet, simple, and genuinely delicious little pud, which is the perfect embodiment of everything a pudding should be, but, sadly, so reviled and sorely neglected. Delicious hot with lots of custard, I also like it cold, straight from the fridge, when it's like a cross between a fruit bun and lardy cake.

There's no need to steam the pudding (this also applies to other suet puddings – jam roly poly, for instance) when baking takes a lot less time; just loosely cover the pudding with foil and put it in the oven. On the other hand, steaming gives the pudding a softer texture all through, whereas baking makes a crust around the outside, so if you want to steam it, wrap the pudding in a double layer of greaseproof inside an old, clean tea towel and pull it into a crescent shape so it fits neatly into a large saucepan of boiling water, then steam it gently with the lid on for 1 ½ –2 hours. (To get the pudding out, strain the water out of the saucepan with the lid half on, tip the pudding onto a flat surface and leave to cool for a few minutes before unwrapping.)

3 oz (75 g) white breadcrumbs
3 oz (75 g) self-raising flour
1 tsp baking powder
2 oz (50 g) suet
2 oz (50 g) caster sugar
6 oz (175 g) currants or sultanas
2 fl oz (60 ml) milk
½ lemon, finely grated rind and juice

METHOD

1. Put a large piece of foil on a baking tray (shiny side upwards) and pre-heat the oven to Gas Mark 5 (190°C).
2. Put the breadcrumbs, flour, baking powder, sugar, suet, fruit, lemon rind and juice in a large bowl, mix together and make a well in the centre.
3. Add the milk to the bowl and mix with a knife or tablespoon until the dough starts to come together, then finish pinching the dough together with the fingers of one hand.
4. Turn the dough out onto a floured surface and sprinkle with a little flour before kneading gently for a minute, then shape the smooth dough into a fat roll approximately 6 inches (10–12 cm) long.
5. Place the spotted dick (there, I said it) on the baking tray, cover loosely with another large piece of foil, shiny side

inwards, and bake in the oven, Gas Mark 5 (190°C) for about 45 minutes. Remove the top piece of foil 5 minutes from the end of cooking time if you want the pudding to have a harder, golden crust.

ALSO TRY...

1. STRAWBERRY MERINGUES: Meringue nests filled with fresh strawberries in season (or tinned fruit cocktail, peaches or pears, any time) and topped with Yeo Valley fruit bio live yoghurt.
2. ORANGE CUPS: This was my mum's way of getting us to eat oranges when we were very small. Just cut the oranges in half, segment the fruit with a sharp knife as you would with a grapefruit, then sprinkle with sugar and put a cherry in the middle.
3. BAKED BANANA CUSTARD: Slice bananas in half lengthways, pour over a pint of instant custard, sprinkle with brown sugar and put in a low oven for 20–30 minutes.
4. FRUIT JELLY: Make jelly with a tin of fruit first thing in the morning (when you're already boiling the kettle to make tea or coffee) and use the fruit juice to make the jelly up to 1 pint (500 ml). It should be set and ready to eat by dinnertime.

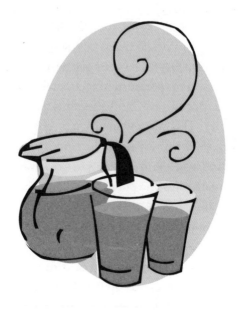

"I don't even butter my bread;
I consider that cooking."

Katherine Cebrian

Can't cook? Don't cook!

However good your intentions, there are bound to be times when even putting toast under the grill seems too much like hard work when all you want to do is eat something and you just can't face another sandwich. Luckily, there are still a few options left...

Tips

Put little bowls of pumpkin and sunflower seeds or monkey nuts out to nibble in front of the television. Children especially enjoy the ritual of peeling and spitting out the shells and are much less likely to eat too many than they would be with salted nuts or crisps.

Breadcrumbs come in handy for so many things, so never throw away the last few slices of a stale loaf; make them into breadcrumbs by cutting the crusts off and whizzing a few slices at a time in the food processor or blender. (As a rough guide, one slice of bread makes about 1 oz (25 g) of breadcrumbs.) If you use very fresh bread, leave the crumbs to dry out on a sheet of greaseproof paper for about half an hour. Mix the remains of different types of bread and store in the freezer in old bread bags.

Buy frozen fruit from the supermarket; (you'll find several variations) it's cheaper than fresh, defrosts very quickly, and is perfect for making ready-chilled fruit and vegetable smoothies.

Readymade coleslaw can be slimy and revolting but packets of fresh coleslaw vegetables are pretty good if you haven't got time to make it from scratch; just add mayonnaise and yoghurt with lemon juice and seasoning at home.

Whether you're very hungry or just peckish, you should be able to find something here to tide you over to the next cooked meal.

Celery sticks cut in half and filled with peanut butter or cream cheese.

Slices of ham spread with soft cheese, rolled up and eaten with chunks of tomato.

Rice cakes spread with peanut butter or cream cheese and slices of cucumber.

Flour or corn tortilla wraps filled with ham, grated cheese and coleslaw ... almost, but not quite a sandwich.

Quickest guacamole: avocados mashed with natural yoghurt, seasoned and served with carrot sticks and tortilla chips.

Smoked mackerel (with lots of lemon juice) and brown bread and butter.

Salad: lettuce, spinach, watercress, mustard & cress, cucumber, tomatoes, radishes, peppers, sweetcorn, grated carrot, celery, avocado, cheese, ham, tuna, salmon, croutons...

Prawn cocktails: Blend a couple of tablespoons of mayonnaise with the same amount of tomato ketchup and mix in the prawns, then spoon them over shredded lettuce, spinach or watercress, sliced cucumber and chunks of avocado. Sprinkle with paprika and crushed up, readymade croutons, if you have them.

Get those leftovers out of the freezer (soup, chilli, spag bol, moussaka, shepherd's pie, lasagne, pasta sauce, fish pie, fish cakes, pancakes...) and re-heat in the microwave. That's not really cooking, is it? No.

SMOOTHIES: The possibilities are endless, so experiment ... or buy a book. Here are a few tried and tested recipes to be getting on with.

THE JAMIE OLIVER: Mix 1 large or 2 small bananas, a generous handful of frozen berries and a glass of apple juice in a blender or food processor; serves four.

THE DR GILLIAN: Infuriating, I know (which, incidentally, is a word many people associate with Gillian McKeith) but you need a juicer for this. Take half a bag of curly kale, wash well and put through the juicer with 2 lemons, cut into quarters. Very refreshing, however bad it sounds – and you **just know** it's doing you good.

THE JANE CLARKE (NUTRITIONIST AND FOOD WRITER): Half a (ripe) mango, 2 tbsp of natural yoghurt and a glass of fresh orange juice, blended.

BANANA SMOOTHIE: 1 large or 2 small bananas, 2 tbsp natural yoghurt, 1 scoop of vanilla ice cream, **1/2** tsp nutmeg, honey (to taste). Peel the bananas and put them in the blender with the rest of the ingredients; adjust the amounts according to taste, blend for 2 minutes and pour into tall glasses with plenty of ice.

CARROT, CELERY AND APPLE: 2–3 carrots, depending on size, a few sticks of celery and a large glass of apple juice, blended on high for a minute.

ISOTONIC DRINK: If you're already addicted to sugary, fizzy, so-called 'sports' drinks, this won't impress you much, but as a healthier and cheaper alternative, it's pretty good, and it does exactly the same job without damaging your teeth or your diet.

THIS FILLS A 500 ML BOTTLE OF WATER (ALMOST 1 PINT):
450 ml of water
50 ml of lemon or lime juice – or 25 ml of each
2 teaspoons of sugar
1 small pinch of salt

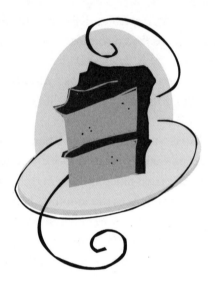

"He who does not mind his belly,
will hardly mind anything else."

Samuel Johnson

Let them eat cake

There can't be many things more disappointing than your average doughnut. Bland, tasteless dough, uncomfortably gritty sugar, a little squirt of jam and it's all over. Even worse, if you get the little squirt of jam in the first mouthful there's nothing to look forward to. What else can you do except eat another one?

Maybe the biggest myth about baking cakes, apart from the idea that it's only for sissies, is that it requires a considerable amount of time, patience and skill when in fact the opposite is true; making your own cakes must be one of the easiest, most therapeutic and rewarding past-times ever. Anyone can do it.

The cakes in this chapter are divided into three sections: things to make with your children just for the fun of it; wholesome cakes full of fruit, bran, oats, nuts and seeds, which are healthy enough to eat for breakfast (although I'm not sure how to square that with the fact that I wouldn't normally eat the cakes in the first section for breakfast, even though some of them contain breakfast cereal); and special occasion cakes for when you have more time and feel like showing off a bit.

What you need

Everything here can be made just as easily in a blender or food processor, but I prefer my old handheld electric whisk because it gives me a bit more control over the whole process and saves on the washing up. The only other things you need are a large mixing bowl, metal tablespoons, a set of scales or a measuring jug, and a couple of cake tins.

Cake tins

A standard size (1lb) loaf tin is perfect for tea breads. For larger cakes I nearly always use two shallower 7″ (18 cm) sandwich tins instead of one deeper tin; it's easier to judge the cooking time that way and it dispenses with the hassle of cutting a much bigger cake in half if you want to fill it with jam or cream afterwards. Where a recipe requires one cake tin rather than a standard loaf tin or sandwich tins, an 8″ tin (21 cm) – round or square – generally works well, although the one I use at home is actually a rectangular roasting tin with straight sides, roughly 8″ x 10″ (21 cm x 28 cm) and about 1 ½ (3 cm) deep.

You can always use an old biscuit tin instead of a cake tin, the only difference being that a biscuit tin won't be non-stick, so make sure you grease it well and line it completely. Biscuit tins make good substitutes when you want something more unusual – a heart-shaped or octagonal cake, for instance – and you can't find the tin you want in the shops.

Lining the tin

You don't have to fiddle around trying to make little bits of greaseproof paper or baking parchment fit all four sides of the cake tin. A lot of cake recipes tell you to 'base line' the tin, but I like to cut one long piece of greaseproof which goes across the bottom of the tin and up two of the sides, leaving about an inch (2 or 3 cms) of surplus sticking up above the edge. This makes it easy to lift the cake straight out of the tin afterwards; I've called it long-strip-lining in the recipes. For round cakes, draw a circle round the bottom of the tin straight onto the greaseproof paper. If you're using two shallow sandwich tins you won't need to line the sides.

Grease cake tins with a different fat from the one you're using in the cake mixture; for example, if the recipe calls for butter, grease the tin with sunflower oil for a guaranteed non-stick result. Use screwed-up greaseproof paper (or kitchen roll if you're using oil) to grease the bottom and sides of the tin; then line the tin with the greaseproof paper and lightly grease that too.

How to tell when the cake is cooked

Smaller, individual cakes should be soft and springy but firm to the touch. For larger cakes, insert a skewer or a very thin, sharp knife into the middle of the cake; if it comes out clean, the cake is ready. If the cake is cooked on the outside but still a bit gooey on the inside (i.e. the skewer comes out streaked with raw cake mixture) cover the top with a couple of layers of greaseproof paper, or silver foil with the shiny side down to draw more heat towards the inside of the cake.

Putting it in the tin

Plastic spatulas are perfect for scraping the bowl – I keep meaning to get one – but any large spoon will do. For stickier cakes like Flapjacks, use a tablespoon and fork to get the mixture into the tin. Cakes naturally rise in the middle, so spread the mixture towards the sides of the tin and hollow it out slightly in the centre.

Getting it out of the tin

After a minute or two the cake will shrink away from the sides of the tin ever so slightly; run a sharp knife around the edges and gently lift the cake out by holding the greaseproof paper on either side. If you haven't got enough paper to get hold of, place a wire cooling tray over the top of the cake, carefully turn it over and ease the tin away from the cake.

Measuring

You can buy a set of measuring spoons, scales and a measuring jug in any kitchen shop or large supermarket. Lots of the cakes in this chapter don't require the ingredients to be 100 per cent accurate anyway, and even if they do, once you've learnt what an ounce (or 25 g) of flour looks like you'll probably find you can do without a proper measuring tool altogether most of the time.

A heaped tablespoon (or a level serving spoon) = 1 oz / 25 g. Use the same sized spoon every time you measure and you'll soon get the hang of it.

I must admit I still think in ounces, pounds and inches rather than metric, so although you shouldn't have problems using either, there's the tiniest possibility that the imperial measurements will be *slightly* more accurate.

Finally, if you're not sure about size, fill a tin or pudding basin with flour and weigh that; e.g. a 1 lb loaf tin will hold 1 lb of flour.

Approximate weights and measures

SPOONS:

1 teaspoon (1 tsp)................5ml

1 dessert spoon..................10 ml

1 tablespoon (1 tbsp)........15 ml

LIQUID MEASURES:

1 fl oz....................................25 ml

¼ pint (5 fl oz)..................125 ml

DRY WEIGHTS:

½ oz..............................15 g

1 oz..............................25 g

1 ¼ oz..........................40 g

2 oz..............................50 g

3 oz..............................75 g

4 oz (¼ lb)......100−125 g

5 oz..............................150 g

LIQUID MEASURES:

⅓ pint..............................200 ml

½ pint..............................300 ml

¾ pint..............................400 ml

1 pint (20 fl oz)..............600 ml

2 pints.............................1.1 litre

DRY WEIGHTS:

6 oz ....175 g

8 oz (½ lb)................225 g

12 oz (¾ lb)...........350 g

1 lb..............................450 g

1 ¼ lb.......................550 g

1 ½ lb.......................675 g

1 ¾ lb....................800 g

2 lb................900 g–1 kg

For best results

Much as I love a shortcut, I always, *always* sieve the flour; you get a much better result if it's sifted; it only takes a few seconds to push flour through a sieve and a few seconds more to rinse the sieve under the hot tap, so there's no point in skipping it.

Get to know your oven. (If you have a fan oven you may find you have to reduce the temperature in some recipes by about 10 degrees.) Always pre-heat your oven and bake cakes in the middle of the oven, unless otherwise stated in the recipe.

Tips

To 'rub in' flour and fat, use only your fingertips and hold your hands high above the bowl to keep the mixture cool and light.

A niftier way of 'rubbing in' (for some recipes) is to cream the butter and sugar with an electric hand whisk, just long enough to mix the two together (no need to spend time getting it pale and fluffy as you would for a sponge cake), then beat in the flour on the lowest speed setting for a few seconds until the mixture resembles fine breadcrumbs.

If you think a sponge mixture is about to curdle, add 1

teaspoon of flour with each addition of egg.

For an even softer consistency, use icing sugar instead of caster sugar in a sponge recipe.

Make baking powder with 2 parts cream of tartar to 1 part bicarbonate of soda.

Make a good substitute for self-raising flour by adding 1 teaspoon of baking powder to 8 oz (225 g) plain flour.

Keep lemons at room temperature; before squeezing, press and roll them on a hard surface, which makes it easier to extract the juice. (As a rough guide, one large lemon makes approximately 2 tablespoons of juice.)

If you crack eggs straight into the bowl one bad egg can ruin the whole lot, so break them separately into a cup first and add them to the mixture one at a time.

COOKING WITH CHILDREN

I worked with primary school children for years when my own children were small and I never came across a single one, boy or girl, who didn't enjoy cooking as an activity. The downside of your children baking at school, especially with the very young ones, is you never know whose sticky little fingers have been where; anything can happen between the mixing bowl, the oven and beyond, even if they've all been made to wash their hands first. (It's hard not to think about these things sometimes.) My elder son never failed to save me a nice big piece of whatever it was he made when he was little, so when his younger brother came along and kept his cakes all to himself without offering me so much as a bite ... I breathed a huge sigh of relief.

At least when you're cooking at home you have a bit more control in the hygiene department, and anything you can do with a class of twenty-five has to be easier in your own kitchen with only two or three children.

One of the great advantages of cooking with children of all ages, apart from getting them interested in food, is that doing something together in the kitchen creates a perfect, informal opportunity to talk, which can otherwise be quite hard to come by in the average household where everyone constantly rushes off in different directions all the time.

Not only that, if you get them interested early on, by the time your kids are teenagers they should be able to produce the occasional family meal themselves ... although that probably won't include doing the washing up.

EASY CHEESY BISCUITS

You'll find very cheap sets of biscuit cutters shaped like animals, teddies, stars and so on in most toy stores, as well as supermarkets and kitchen shops. Buy at least two different sets; once you've got them you'll be using them forever.

The thinner you roll out the dough, the crisper these biscuits will be, so cut them out in varying thicknesses until you find out which way you like them best, or do some thick, some thin.

(Leave out the egg yolk if you like, it doesn't make a lot of difference – ditto the paprika.)

VARIABLE AMOUNT, DEPENDING ON SIZE OF CUTTER, THICKNESS OF DOUGH...
4 oz (100 g) plain flour
2 oz (50 g) butter or margarine
2 oz (50 g) cheese
Splash of milk
1 egg yolk
1 tsp paprika

METHOD

1. Sieve the flour and paprika into a large mixing bowl; add the butter or margarine in little pieces and rub in with your fingertips until the mixture resembles rough breadcrumbs.
2. Add the grated cheese, stir, then make a well in the centre, pour in the milk and egg yolk and mix it all together to make a firm dough.
3. Put the dough on a floured surface and knead it for a bit, then divide the pastry into two pieces, wrap one half in clingfilm and keep it in the fridge while you roll out the other half.
4. Cut the biscuits out, place on lightly greased oven trays and bake on Gas Mark 5 (190°C) for 10 –15 minutes, until the biscuits are a light golden brown.

CHEESE & COURGETTE SCONES

Any recipe for scones is very simple for children to make and these are much nicer than they sound, so don't be put off if you're not used to the idea of making cakes and biscuits with grated vegetables; once upon a time we thought carrot cake was on the weird side; now it's as normal and accepted as a jam tart (see below.)

Traditionally, scones tend to be made with plain flour, cream of tartar, and bicarbonate of soda, but self-raising flour alone works brilliantly – and you don't need a rolling pin either; just pummel the dough out roughly with your hands, cut out the scones, then knead the remains together again, repeating the process until you run out of dough.

To make fruit scones, mix a couple of tablespoons of sugar and a handful of sultanas (washed in warm water) with the rubbed-in flour and butter before adding the milk.

MAKES ABOUT 12:
8 oz (225 g) self-raising flour
Salt & pepper
2 oz (50 g) butter or margarine
2 ½ fl oz (60 ml) milk
2 oz (50 g) grated cheddar cheese
1 courgette, peeled and grated

METHOD
1. Sift the flour and seasoning into a large mixing bowl.
2. Grate the cheese and courgette together on a dinner plate.
3. Add the butter in small pieces to the flour in the mixing bowl, rub in with your fingertips until the mixture resembles medium-fine breadcrumbs, and make a well in the centre.
4. Add the milk, grated cheese and courgette, and mix it all together to make a soft dough.
5. Turn the dough onto a floured surface and knead for a minute, then press out to about 1 inch thickness and cut into rounds with a pastry cutter, tumbler, or cup.
6. Place the scones on a greased baking tray about an inch (2 cm) apart, glaze with milk and bake on Gas Mark 7 (220°C) for about 10 minutes, until the scones are risen and light golden brown on top.

JAM TARTS

Yet another recipe where you only need approximate measurements, but if you want to weigh out the ingredients as part of the activity, just roughly translate the number of tablespoons into ounces or grammes.

MAKES 12 (OR 18 MINIS) DEPENDING ON THE SIZE OF THE PASTRY CUTTER:

4 tbsp plain flour

2 tbsp butter

1 tbsp sugar

2 tbsp milk

Jam, marmalade or lemon curd

Milk for glazing

METHOD

1. Sift the flour into a mixing bowl and rub in the butter until the mixture resembles medium-fine breadcrumbs.
2. Stir in the sugar, then add the milk and mix together to make a firm dough.
3. Turn the dough onto a floured surface and roll it out to about 1mm thick.
4. Cut out rounds with a pastry cutter – or any cup that looks about the right size for the job – and place them in a greased bun tin.
5. Glaze each pastry circle with a little milk, then prick twice with a fork and put a teaspoon of jam in each one. (Don't overfill as the jam expands in the oven.)
6. Bake on Gas Mark 5 (190°C) for about 10 minutes, or until the pastry is a light, golden brown.

CHOCOLATE RICE KRISPIE CAKES

The favourite of old favourites; add mini marshmallows or brightly coloured hundreds and thousands to make them more interesting – or raisins if you're desperately trying to get your children to eat more fruit. (Even if they usually pick the pieces of fruit out of everything, it's always possible that they might eat some by mistake.)

MAKES APPROXIMATELY 24 CAKES:
2 x 4 oz (110 g) bars of milk chocolate
Rice Krispies

METHOD
1. Melt the chocolate in a bowl over a saucepan of boiling water.
2. Stir in the Rice Krispies; as many as possible, making sure they're all well covered in chocolate.
3. Spoon the mixture into cake cases and leave to set for about an hour. (If it's very hot, keep them in the fridge.)

CORNFLAKE CAKES

1 x 4 oz (110 g) bar of milk or plain chocolate
2 heaped tbsp golden syrup
2 oz (50 g) butter or margarine
4 oz (100 g) cornflakes
1 oz (25 g) desiccated coconut

METHOD
1. Melt the butter, syrup and chocolate in a bowl over a saucepan of boiling water.
2. Add the cornflakes and coconut and mix well.
3. Spoon into cake cases and leave to set for at least an hour. (As with Krispie cakes, store them in the fridge if it's hot.)

FAIRY CAKES

There's no end to what you can use for decorating fairy cakes; Smarties, chocolate buttons, jelly beans, hundreds and thousands, glace cherries, walnuts ... or just use piping gel to make patterns on the icing.

Make butterfly cakes by cutting out a circle of sponge from the centre of each cake, filling the holes with butter icing, then cutting the circles in half and placing them on top of the butter icing to look like wings. Finish by dusting with a little icing sugar.

To make chocolate fairy cakes, substitute 1 oz (25 g) of cocoa powder for about 1 oz (25 g) of the flour.

To make a Victoria sponge, grease and base line two 7″ (18 cm) sandwich tins and increase the quantities of the basic mixture by half, i.e. 6 oz (150g) each of flour, butter and sugar, and three eggs.

MAKES ABOUT 24 CAKES:
4 oz (100 g) self-raising flour
4 oz (100 g) butter or margarine
4 oz (100 g) sugar
2 eggs, beaten

METHOD
1. Cream the butter and sugar in a large mixing bowl until pale and fluffy (takes about 3 minutes with an electric hand whisk).
2. Gradually add the beaten egg to the mixture a little at a time and keep whisking. If the mixture starts to curdle, i.e. it looks lumpy and holey, a bit like cellulite (not your cellulite, someone else's), throw in a teaspoonful of the flour with each addition of egg.
3. Fold in the flour with a large spoon, making sure you've got it all in.
4. Spoon the mixture into cake cases and bake in the oven, Gas Mark 5 (190°C) for 10–15 minutes; the sponges should be a light golden colour and firm and springy to the touch.

ICING FAIRY CAKES
BUTTER ICING: *Roughly 1 part butter or margarine to 3 parts icing sugar.*

1. Sieve the icing sugar into a large bowl with the butter; add 2 tablespoons of hot water and beat it all together. Use a couple of drops of food colouring if you like, and if you think the icing is still too thick, add a little more hot water a drop at a time until you get the consistency you want.

GLACE ICING: *Roughly 1 tablespoon of water to 4 tablespoons of icing sugar.*
1. Sieve the icing sugar into a large bowl and add a *little lukewarm water very gradually*, stirring all the time. Glace icing can go from too stodgy to pure liquid in seconds, so work slowly, but don't worry if you end up with runny icing; just sieve some more icing sugar in until you've got it the way you want.

GINGERBREAD MEN

Again, measurements don't need to be exact – but don't be tempted to overdo the golden syrup or the dough will become too soft and unworkable.

(Store in a tin with a tight-fitting lid to stop the gingerbread men jumping out and running away.)

MAKES ABOUT 12 LARGE GINGERBREAD MEN:
6 tbsp (6 oz /175 g) plain flour
½ tsp bicarbonate of soda
2 tsp ginger
Pinch of salt
2 tbsp (2 oz/50 g) butter or margarine
3 tbsp (3 oz/85 g) soft brown sugar
1 egg
1 tbsp golden syrup
Currants

METHOD

1. Grease two baking trays and pre-heat the oven to Gas Mark 4/5 (180/190°C).
2. Wash a big handful of currants in a sieve and leave them to drain on kitchen roll or an old, clean tea towel.
3. Sift the dry ingredients into a large mixing bowl: flour, bicarbonate of soda, salt and ginger.
4. Rub in the butter with your fingertips to make rough breadcrumbs.
5. Mix in the sugar and make a well in the centre.
6. Put the egg and golden syrup into the well and use a fork to stir everything together to make a soft, pliable dough.
7. Turn the dough out onto a floured surface, knead for a minute until it feels ready, then roll out to about 1/8″ (3 mm) thickness.
8. Cut out as many gingerbread men as you can and place them on the baking trays, then roll out the remaining dough and cut out more. Keep going until you've run out of dough.
9. Press currants firmly onto the gingerbread men where you want their eyes, mouths and buttons to be.
10. Bake in the centre and/or the top of the oven on Gas Mark 4–5 (180/190°C) for 10–15 minutes, until the gingerbread men are crisp and golden.

SWEETLOAF

I wouldn't recommend using cooking chocolate for this – in fact I wouldn't recommend using cooking chocolate for anything – but a mixture of 'better' chocolate (i.e. Cadbury's, Galaxy or supermarket own brand) with SOME cooking chocolate would probably be okay. Malted milk or rich tea biscuits are perfect, but digestives, Penguins or Viscount Biscuits work equally well. Chopped hazelnuts and glace cherries are also good, so use them instead of the marshmallows if you prefer – if you want nuts and cherries in addition to the marshmallows, reduce the amount of biscuits.

For a grown-up version, make the sweetloaf with the best chocolate you can get your hands on and cut it into super-thin slithers at the end. It should look (and taste) good enough to give to guests with the coffee after dinner.

Approx 1 ½ lb (1 kg) milk chocolate
4 oz (100 g) unsalted butter
8 rich tea or malted milk biscuits
4 ginger biscuits
A generous handful each of mini marshmallows and raisins

METHOD
1. *Very lightly grease* and long-strip-line a standard (1 lb) loaf tin.
2. Break the chocolate into small pieces and put it in a bowl over a pan of boiling water to melt.
3. Melt the butter separately – in the microwave is good; about 40 seconds on 'defrost' – and never be tempted to try and melt the butter and chocolate together for this; for some reason it just turns into a thick, lumpy, unworkable mess.
4. Wash and dry the raisins; break up the biscuits on a dinner plate or in a bowl; add the dried fruit and marshmallows and mix it all up together.
5. When the chocolate has melted, stir in the melted butter followed by the rest of the ingredients and pour the mixture into the lined loaf tin.
6. Leave to chill in the fridge for several hours, preferably overnight; cut into very thin slices and serve. (N.B. *The colder and harder the sweetloaf becomes, the easier it is to cut into super-thin slithers,*

which is why it's worth keeping it in the fridge for longer. Otherwise, cut thicker slices, then cut the slices into fingers.)

TREACLE CRUNCHES

I love these; black treacle is a good source of iron and there's no added sugar, so I like to think they're a slightly healthier option than some of the other cakes in this section.

MAKES ABOUT 18:
½ lb (approx 225 g) milk chocolate
1 heaped tbsp black treacle
8 oz (220 g) digestive biscuits (roughly 16 biscuits)
4 oz (100 g) butter or margarine

METHOD
1. Crumble the digestive biscuits into tiny pieces (use your hands, or bash them up with a heavy object; a mug or a rolling pin will do) and break the chocolate into squares.
2. Melt the butter first in a bowl over a saucepan of boiling water, then add the black treacle.
3. Add the chocolate to the bowl and stir for a minute or two until it's thoroughly melted and there are no lumps left.
4. Mix the broken biscuits into the chocolate, then spoon the mixture into cake cases and leave to set in the fridge for about an hour.

CHOCOLATE CHIP COOKIES

You can buy chocolate chips in the baking section at the supermarket, but these are more fun if you use Smarties and crush them up yourself by putting them in a plastic food bag, or something similar, and bashing them with a cup or rolling pin.

MAKES ABOUT 24 BISCUITS:

8 oz (225 g) self-raising flour

5 oz (150 g) butter or margarine

4 oz (100 g) caster sugar

1 egg, beaten

2 oz (50 g) broken Smarties or chocolate chips

METHOD

1. Sift the flour into a large mixing bowl, add the butter or margarine in small pieces and rub in until the mixture resembles medium-fine breadcrumbs.
2. Stir in the sugar then make a well in the centre, add the beaten egg and mix to a stiff dough.
3. Turn the dough onto a floured surface and knead for a couple of minutes until smooth, then work in the Smarties or chocolate chips, wrap the dough in clingfilm or foil and chill in the fridge for 30 minutes.
4. Roll out the chilled dough to about 1/8″ thick (3 mm) and cut out biscuits with a pastry cutter, cup or beaker.
5. Place the biscuits a little way apart on greased baking sheets, prick them with a fork a few times, and bake on Gas Mark 4 (180°C) for about 10 minutes, until golden.

WHOLESOME CAKES

No matter how sugary, scrumptious and inviting a shop-bought cake appears to be on the outside, the instant you bite into it you realise how unappetising it is, whereas, what these wholesome cakes may lack in the looks department, they more than make up for in taste, texture, and the sheer enjoyment of eating something sweet that's actually quite good for you.

CARROT CAKE

There are lots of methods for making carrot cake. I think this is probably the easiest and the result is a lovely moist cake that keeps in the fridge for a few days, assuming it's around that long. I use Quark, the virtually fat-free soft cheese for the topping, but you can use any other low-fat cream cheese, or even full-fat cream cheese if you prefer, it doesn't make much difference to the end result either way.

FOR THE CAKE:
8 oz (225 g) self-raising flour
8 oz (225 g) soft brown sugar
8 oz (225 g) butter
4 eggs – whites and yolks separated
1 tsp baking powder
5 small or 3 large carrots
1 orange
1 lemon

FOR THE TOPPING:
8 oz (225 g) tub of cream cheese or Quark
3 tbsp runny honey
orange/lemon juice

OPTIONAL:
5 oz (150 g) walnuts – broken into small pieces

METHOD
1. Grease and line the bottom of two 7″ (18 cm) sandwich tins with greaseproof paper or baking parchment. Pre-heat oven to Gas Mark 4 (180°C).

2. Wash and cut the orange and lemon in half; put the finely grated rind of half the orange into a small bowl with the juice, plus the juice of one of the lemon halves. (Put the remaining halves of orange and lemon aside for the topping.)
3. Cream butter and sugar in a large mixing bowl until pale and fluffy.
4. Beat in the eggs yolks and then add the lemon/orange juice and rind.
5. Fold in the flour and baking powder
6. Whisk the egg whites till stiff and smooth-looking (all the bubbles will disappear) and fold into the cake mixture, followed by the grated carrots – and the walnut pieces if you're using them.
7. Divide the mixture equally between the prepared tins and bake in a moderate oven for about 45 minutes.
8. When the cakes are cool, beat the honey and cream cheese together with the remainder of the orange and lemon juice. Use half to sandwich the cakes together and spread the rest on the top.

BRAN LOAF

More delicious than shop-bought malt loaf and so easy to fling together a child can do it. This must be one of the only cake mixtures that looks and tastes pretty revolting in the bowl, but honestly, the end result is well worth the complete lack of effort...

Best sliced thinly and eaten with butter or jam.

1 mug of Kellogg's All-Bran
1 mug of either currants, mixed dried fruit, or sultanas
1 mug of milk
1 mug of self-raising flour
A generous half-mug of caster or soft brown sugar

METHOD

1. Put everything except the flour in a large bowl and leave the mixture to stand for about an hour.
2. Grease and long-strip-line a standard size loaf tin and pre-heat the oven to approximately Gas Mark 3 (160°C).
3. Sift the flour into the soggy mixture; stir it in well and pour the whole lot into the loaf tin, spreading it evenly up to the sides.
4. Bake in a cool oven for about an hour and a half, until a skewer or sharp knife inserted into the middle of the cake comes out clean.

ROCK BUNS

These aren't much like the rock cakes I've found in the supermarket, which were pale and flat with only about 3 sultanas in each one. I use more fruit, slightly less fat and *a lot* less sugar than I've found in other recipes, but these rock cakes are as good as any I've eaten – and I've got a sweet tooth. I like to use soft brown sugar, but there's no reason why you can't use demerara, caster, or just plain granulated if that's all you've got.

MAKES ABOUT 24 BUNS:

1 lb (450 g) self-raising flour
6 oz (150 g) butter or margarine
2 oz (50 g) soft brown sugar
2 eggs
1 lb (450 g) bag of dried fruit
A big splash of milk
1 tsp nutmeg
1 tsp cinnamon
1 tsp mixed spice

METHOD

1 Grease two baking sheets and pre-heat oven to Gas Mark 6 (200°C). Wash the fruit in warm water and assemble the rest of the ingredients.

2. Sift the flour into a very large mixing bowl and rub in the butter or margarine in small pieces.

3. Don't over-work the mixture; as soon as it vaguely resembles rough breadcrumbs, add the sugar, spices and fruit and mix it all together.

4. Make a well in the centre and pour in the beaten eggs with a big of splash of milk, then gradually work the liquid into the mixture to make a stiff, moist, dough, adding another splash of milk if you think the mixture is too dry.

5. Using a dessert spoon and your fingers, shape the mixture into rocky lumps (roughly the size of ping-pong balls) on the greased baking sheets, and bake in the oven for about 20 minutes until they're a light, golden brown.

GINGER CAKE

Ginger cakes are always best left for a couple days before eating (some recipes recommend waiting a whole week!), which gives them time to develop that lovely soft, sticky texture. If you haven't got black treacle, use twice the amount of golden syrup; the end result will still be good, but a bit lighter in colour and texture.

4 oz (100 g) golden syrup
and
4 oz (100 g) black treacle
or 8 oz (225 g) golden syrup

8 oz (225 g) plain flour
¼ tsp bicarbonate of soda
1 tsp mixed spice
2 oz (50 g) butter
2 oz (50 g) lard
1 tsp ginger
4 oz (100 g) soft dark brown sugar
A very little milk

METHOD
1. Put the syrup and treacle in a small saucepan with the butter and lard on a very low heat while you assemble the rest of the ingredients and long-strip-line a square cake tin. Pre-heat the oven to Gas Mark 3 (170°C) or slightly lower; this takes over an hour to cook and you don't want it to burn.
2. Sift the flour and bicarbonate of soda into a large bowl with the sugar and spices, mix everything together and make a well in the centre.
3. Pour the melted fat and syrup/treacle mixture into the centre.
4. Beat the mixture well, starting in the centre and working outwards to incorporate all the dry ingredients, adding just enough milk to make a thick, smooth batter.
5. Scoop the batter into the cake tin and bake near the bottom of the oven for 1–1 ½ hours until the cake is firm and dark brown.
6. Allow the cake to cool on a wire cooling rack, then wrap it up well in greaseproof paper and foil, or store in an airtight tin for a couple of days.

BANANA CAKE

You can also make banana cake by following the recipe for a basic Victoria sponge *(see Fairy cakes earlier in this chapter)*; just use brown sugar instead of white and add the mashed bananas to the mixture after you've folded in the flour. There's not much to choose between these two methods, except this one uses less butter and sugar, making the end result a bit lighter in texture and slightly less rich.

8 oz (225 g) self-raising flour
4 oz (100 g) butter
4 oz (100 g) dark brown sugar
3–4 bananas, depending on size (mashed)
2 eggs
A very little milk

METHOD
1. Grease and long-strip-line a square cake tin (or a loaf tin, although the top of the cake may split slightly in the standard 1lb size).
2. Gently rub in the butter and flour in a large bowl, using your fingertips and being careful not to over-work the mixture.
3. Stir in the sugar.
4. Add the eggs and the mashed bananas, beating well and adding a little milk to make a soft dropping consistency.
5. Bake on Gas Mark 4 (180°C) for about 45 minutes.

ALL-IN-ONE APPLE CAKE

I once met someone who told me she used to eat whole, raw cake mixtures before she could get them into the tin. I don't think I could, but if I was ever going to be tempted by an uncooked cake mixture, it would have to be this one.

6 oz (15 0g) self-raising flour
1 level tsp baking powder
4 oz (100 g) brown sugar
4 fl oz (100 ml) sunflower oil
2 eggs
5–6 sweet apples (not cooking apples)
4 tsp cinnamon
1 tsp mixed spice

METHOD
1. Grease and line the cake or loaf tin *with butter or margarine* and pre-heat the oven to Gas Mark 5 (190°C).
2. Cut the apples into quarters (or smaller) one at a time, peeling and removing the core and skin, then slicing into small, fine chunks.
3. Mix the prepared apples with the sugar and spices – setting aside a few pieces to stick into the top of the cake, if you like.
4. Sieve the flour and baking powder into a large bowl, make a well in the centre; add the sunflower oil, eggs, and the spiced apples in no particular order, then beat the whole lot together on high speed for half a minute.
5. Pour the mixture into the tin and gently press the reserved pieces of apple into the top. Bake until a skewer inserted into the middle of the cake comes out clean – approximately 40 minutes.

BREAD PUDDING

Make bread pudding in a square 8″ x 8″ (21 cm x 21 cm) cake tin or Pyrex roasting dish; as long as you grease and long-strip-line it properly, either one will do.

1 pint (500 ml) of cold tea and 1 teabag (if you're using a milder
   tea, use 2 teabags)
8 slices of bread from a large, white medium-sliced loaf
8 oz sultanas (half a 500g bag)
4 oz (100 g) brown sugar
1 egg
2 teaspoons mixed spice

METHOD
1. Break the bread into tiny pieces with your hands (you don't
   need to remove the crusts if you're using soft sliced bread) and
   put in a bowl with the cold tea. Mash the bread up well with a
   fork and leave it to stand for at least 10 minutes.
2. Mash again; add the fruit, beaten egg, sugar and spice, and mix it
   all up. (The mixture should be nice and stodgy, but not too soggy.)
3. Put the mixture in the prepared tin, press down well and bake
   in a moderate oven, Gas Mark 5 (190°C) for about 30 minutes
   until the cake is dark brown and firm to the touch. While it's
   cooling, sprinkle the top of the cake with a teaspoonful of
   caster sugar.

FLAPJACKS

Flapjack recipes generally contain added sugar, but with so much
syrup in the mixture I don't think you need it, especially if you
include the dried fruit.

MAKES APPROXIMATELY 16 SMALL SQUARES:
12 heaped tbsp porridge oats
6 oz (150 g) butter
6 tbsp golden syrup

OPTIONAL:

2 tbsp dried fruit, chopped; apricots, dates, sultanas...

METHOD

1. Grease and long-strip-line a 7″ (18 cm) square tin and pre-heat oven to Gas Mark 3 (160°C).
2. Melt the butter and syrup in a pan on the stove and put the porridge oats in a large mixing bowl.
3. Pour the melted butter and syrup over the oats and mix together thoroughly (adding the dried fruit at this stage, if using) and making sure there are no dry lumps of oats hiding in the middle of the mixture.
4. Press the mixture firmly into the tin, using the back of a fork to even it out, and bake in a cool oven, Gas Mark 3 (160°C) for about 20 minutes.
5. Leave the flapjacks to cool for 10 minutes, then mark them into squares or slices with a sharp knife and lift the whole lot out of the tin, using the greaseproof paper.
6. After 40–45 minutes, cut the flapjacks up, then separate and leave to cool completely on a wire tray.

SEED CAKE

This is a very old recipe; the sort of thing your great-granny would have made between putting a week's-worth of washing through the mangle and making dinner for 13 children. Perhaps this isn't quite as wholesome as some of the other cakes in this section, but caraway seeds are good for the digestion apparently, and if all else failed I'd sooner give a child a piece of homemade sponge than a cereal bar for breakfast.

Caraway seeds are slightly bitter, so although the vanilla extract isn't vital, putting it in will give the cake that little bit of added sweetness and flavour it needs.

6 oz (175 g) butter or margarine
6 oz (175 g) caster sugar
3 eggs, beaten
4 oz (100 g) plain flour
4 oz (100 g) self-raising flour
2 tsp caraway seeds
Vanilla extract, 1–2 tsp, according to taste
Splash of milk

METHOD

1. Grease and *completely* line a 7″–8″ (18–21 cm) round cake tin and pre-heat the oven to Gas Mark 3/4 (170/180°C).
2. Beat the butter, sugar and vanilla extract together in a large mixing bowl until pale and fluffy.
3. Add the beaten eggs a little at a time, beating constantly to prevent curdling.
4. Fold in the flour and caraway seeds with a large metal spoon and add a splash of milk to get the mixture to a soft dropping consistency.
5. Scoop the mixture into the prepared tin and bake in the lower-middle half of the oven on Gas Mark 3/4 (170/180°C) for 1 hour. Test the cake with a skewer or sharp, thin-bladed knife to see if it's ready; if the cake is cooked on the outside but still a bit gooey in the middle, put it back in the oven with a big piece of foil or greaseproof paper folded in four over the top to allow the cake to finish cooking without burning.

PLUM CAKE

This is a lovely cake with a soft texture and not too much sugar – even less if you use prunes in natural juice instead of syrup – so dust it with a couple of teaspoons of icing sugar at the end if you like; it still counts as a wholesome cake in this book.

7 oz (175 g) self-raising flour
1 heaped tsp baking powder
4 oz (100 g) soft brown sugar
6 oz (150 g) butter or margarine
2 eggs, beaten
1 tsp mixed spice
1 standard size tin of prunes in syrup or natural juice

METHOD

1. Pre-heat oven to Gas Mark 4 (180°C), grease and long-strip-line a 7″ (18 cm) square cake tin.
2. Empty the tin of prunes into a bowl with the juice or syrup, split the prunes lengthways and remove the stones.
3. Sift the flour, baking powder and mixed spice together.
4. Cream the butter and sugar in a large bowl until pale and fluffy and gradually add the beaten egg with a teaspoon of flour each time to stop the mixture curdling.
5. Add the prunes with the juice or syrup and blend on the slowest setting for just a few seconds to mix everything together without breaking up the fruit too much.
6. Fold in the flour with a large spoon, making sure it's completely incorporated, then scoop the mixture into the prepared cake tin.
7. Bake in the middle of the oven on Gas Mark 4 (180°C) for 30 minutes, or until a skewer or sharp knife comes out clean, then lift the cake out of the tin and leave to cool.

ALMOND & APRICOT MUFFINS

Unlike creamed sponge cakes, muffins don't need to be beaten to a super-smooth batter, so fold the butter and eggs in gently – just enough to get everything loosely combined – and try not to overwork the mixture.

Use whichever kind of dried fruit you want for these; the amounts don't have to be exact. There's no reason why you can't make muffins with fresh fruit either – blueberries and raspberries are ideal – but because I find blueberries too expensive unless they're on special offer, when I do buy them I always feel as if I ought to chew each one 32 times instead of squandering them in cake recipes.

If you do use fresh fruit and it's dripping in juice, gently strain off some of the liquid without pulping the fruit to mush, and reduce the amount of milk to prevent the mixture from ending up too soggy.

Finally, if you don't have muffin cases to hand, ordinary paper cake cases will do.

MAKES 16 – 24 DEPENDING ON SIZE:
8 oz (225 g) plain flour
2 tsp baking powder
½ tsp bicarbonate of soda
1 tsp salt
4 oz (100 g) butter, melted
4 oz (100 g) caster sugar
1 large egg
4 fl oz (125 ml) milk
4 oz (100 g) dried apricots, finely chopped
2 oz (50 g) flaked almonds, broken up

METHOD
1. Melt the butter and leave to one side to cool.
2. Pour the milk into a measuring jug, add the egg and whisk together with a fork.
3. Into a large mixing bowl, sift the flour, baking powder, salt and bicarbonate of soda and add the sugar, chopped apricots and

broken almonds.

4. Make a well in the centre, add the melted butter, egg and milk and mix the whole lot together as sloppily as you like, for a lumpy, uneven mixture.

5. Spoon the mixture into the muffin or cake cases and bake on Gas Mark 5 (190°C) for 10–12 minutes.

MUESLI MUFFINS

If you use completely unsweetened muesli you may want to add an extra tablespoon (1 oz or 25 g) of soft brown sugar.

MAKES 16–24 DEPENDING ON SIZE, I.E. IF USING MUFFIN CASES OR REGULAR CAKE CASES:
8 oz (225 g) plain wholemeal flour
2 tsp baking powder
½ tsp bicarbonate of soda
1 tsp salt
1 tsp mixed spice
1 tsp cinnamon
4 oz (100 g) butter, melted
4 oz (100 g) soft brown sugar
1 large egg
4 fl oz (125 ml) milk
1 mug of muesli

METHOD
1. Melt the butter and leave to one side to cool.
2. Measure the milk in a mixing jug, add the eggs and whisk together with a fork.
3. Into a large mixing bowl, sift the flour, baking powder, bicarbonate of soda, salt and spices (tipping the grains from the

flour back into the bowl afterwards) and add the sugar and muesli.

4. Make a well in the centre, add the melted butter, egg and milk and mix the whole lot together as sloppily as you like, for a lumpy, uneven mixture.

5. Spoon the mixture into the cases and bake in the middle of the oven, Gas Mark 5 (190°C) for 10–12 minutes.

PUMPKIN MUFFINS

This is the same method as the other two muffin recipes *(see above.)* It's hard to give an exact quantity for the pumpkin; everyone's estimation of size differs wildly, as we know, so grate the pumpkin before you start; be careful when you're adding it to the mixture and leave some out if you think you've got too much.

MAKES 16–24 DEPENDING ON SIZE, I.E. IF USING MUFFIN CASES OR REGULAR CAKE CASES:

8 oz (225 g) plain flour
2 tsp baking powder
½ tsp bicarbonate of soda
1 tsp salt
4 oz (100 g) butter, melted
4 oz (100 g) caster sugar
1 large egg
4 fl oz (125 ml) milk
½ small pumpkin
1–2 tbsp crushed pumpkin seeds

METHOD

1. Melt the butter and leave to one side to cool.
2. Pour the milk into a measuring jug, add the egg and whisk together with a fork.

3. Into a large mixing bowl, sift the flour, baking powder, salt and bicarbonate of soda, then add the sugar and give it a good stir.
4. Make a well in the centre, add the melted butter, egg and milk and mix the whole lot together just a little before carefully adding the grated pumpkin and loosely combining to a lumpy, uneven mixture.
5. Add the crushed pumpkin seeds to the mixture, or add some and save the rest for the top of the muffins.
6. Spoon the mixture into the muffin or cake cases, sprinkle the crushed seeds, and bake on Gas Mark 5 (190°C) for 10–12 minutes.

SPECIAL CAKES

Maximum effect for minimum effort; that's what you want when you're making a cake for a special occasion. Even though the end result should look pretty spectacular, all the cakes in this section are easily achievable, or they wouldn't be in this book. Trust me.

SWISS ROLL

A Swiss roll is very straightforward to make, contains only a very few cheap ingredients and can easily be turned into something special; a chocolate log at Christmas or a Caterpillar birthday cake, for instance. There's no butter in the mixture either so if you fill your Swiss roll with jam and/or a low fat-free cream cheese instead of double cream, it's pretty low in calories too.

Make Swiss rolls in a standard size baking tray (the one I use is 15″ x 11″ x 1″) and line the tin *completely* so the greaseproof paper comes about an inch (2 cm) above all four sides of the tin, then snip out the corners so there aren't any little folds of paper left to get stuck into the cake mixture, making the greaseproof paper impossible to get off without tearing the sponge, once it's cooked.

3 eggs
4oz caster sugar
4oz plain flour
2 tbsp hot water

METHOD
TO MAKE A CHOCOLATE SWISS ROLL:
Instead of 4 oz (100 g) flour, use 3 oz (75 g) flour and 1 oz (25 g) of cocoa powder. If you don't have cocoa powder, you can use drinking chocolate instead; the texture of the cake will be more or less the same, although it won't have anything like as good a colour or flavour.

1. Grease and line the tin as described above; pre-heat the oven to Gas Mark 6 (200°C).
2. Whisk the eggs and sugar in a bowl until the mixture is thick, pale and creamy and more or less double in size. This takes between 5 and 10 minutes, depending on the type of whisk or blender you're using. (Don't even attempt to do this by hand unless you're supernaturally strong with the patience of a saint.)
3. Gently fold half the flour into the mixture (or flour + cocoa if you're making chocolate), followed by the hot water, then the rest of the flour, taking care not to beat the mixture; it should be a soft, smooth dropping consistency.
4. Scrape the batter into the tin, tilting the tin to help spread the mixture evenly.
5. Bake in a hot oven, Gas Mark 6 (200°C) for about 10 minutes until the sponge is risen, slightly golden and springy to the touch. This cake cooks quickly, so don't go off and do something else; get ready for the next stage.

ROLLING IT UP:

1. Wet a tea towel (an old, thin, threadbare one works best) then tightly wring it out so it's only slightly damp and put it on a clean surface. Lay a clean sheet of greaseproof paper (at least a couple of inches bigger than the cake) on top of the damp tea towel and sprinkle it with sugar.

2. Turn the cooked Swiss roll out onto the clean, sugared greaseproof paper and carefully peel off the old paper from the bottom of the cake.

3. Working as quickly as you can without tying yourself up in knots, trim the crusty edges off the cake, if there are any. Now flip the greaseproof paper over the short end of the sponge nearest to you; start with a tight fold and gently but firmly roll the whole thing up with the greaseproof paper and damp cloth inside, then leave to cool for about half an hour.

TO FILL WITH JAM OR LEMON CURD:

You can do this while the cake is still warm, so have the jam or lemon curd ready when the cake comes out of the oven; spread it over the warm cake as soon as you've peeled the greaseproof paper off, then roll the cake up in the usual way.

TO FILL WITH CREAM:

If you're filling the Swiss roll with butter cream, fresh cream, or a combination of jam and cream, roll the cake up in the way described above; then when it's cool, carefully unroll the cake – you don't need to flatten it out completely – spread the filling over the cake and roll it back up without the greaseproof paper and tea towel.

CATERPILLAR CAKE

There's more than one way of icing a caterpillar cake, so use the suggestions below as a rough guide – you'll probably come up with better ideas of your own. Unless you're one of those mums so brilliant at cake decorating she could give up the day job and turn professional, it's a good idea to make your kids a novelty cake when they're still young and uncritical enough to appreciate your efforts. If your finished caterpillar isn't as good looking as you hoped it would be, pretend it's a worm that's just crawled out of the earth, put it on a plate and surround it with Rice Krispie cakes *(see Cooking With Children earlier in this chapter)*.

FOR A GREEN CATERPILLAR:
Swiss roll (see recipe above)
Glace icing (see page 177)
Green food colouring
Liquorice Allsorts
Chocolate buttons
Chocolate marshmallow teacakes

METHOD
1. Make glace icing in the usual way *(see notes, page 177)* and add 1 or 2 drops of colouring to get the shade you want. Keep the icing on the thin side so you can pour and spread it over the Swiss roll easily; if it's a bit too thin and you can see the cake through it, wait for the icing to dry, then make more icing and repeat the process. *I'd transfer the caterpillar to the cake board or plate now, rather than risk an accident at the end when the damage will be harder to disguise.*
2. Before the icing has dried completely, stick the chocolate buttons along the caterpillar's back to make little spikes (or

lay them flat, like spots), cut the marshmallows in half and place them at regular intervals along the bottom of the cake, 4 on each side, like little feet, and use 2 of the liquorice cylinders from the Liquorice Allsorts to make the antennae. The pink and yellow Allsorts with a round bit of black liquorice in the middle make good eyes and mouths; use different colours for each and slice them in half if you think they're too thick.

ALTERNATIVES:

For a chocolate caterpillar, make chocolate butter icing or melt cooking chocolate and add a couple of spoonfuls of cream when the chocolate starts cooling. Make the easy chocolate frosting *(see notes, page 204)* or use a readymade chocolate frosting from the baking section at the supermarket, although you might find it's a bit harder to spread all over the cake without making a mess of the sponge.

Use Smarties, Jellytots or mini marshmallows to decorate the caterpillar's back instead of chocolate buttons.

Colour the glacé icing with pink, yellow or orange food colouring.

CHOCOLATE YULE LOG

Rather than have a too-small log, I'd make two and use one to make a branch and add a bit of length to the other, in which case you'd need to double up the quantities below.

3 eggs
4 oz (100 g) caster sugar
3 oz (75 g) plain flour
1 oz (25 g) cocoa powder.

METHOD

1. Leave the Swiss roll as it is, or cut a piece diagonally about 2 inches (4 cm) from one end, which you can attach to the side

of the log with butter icing to make it look like a branch.

2. Make plenty of chocolate butter icing *(see notes, page 176)* to fill and cover the log completely, marking the icing with a fork, to resemble bark.

3. Stick a robin or a snowman, or something similar, on top of the cake, and finish by sprinkling a spoonful of icing sugar through a sieve to look like snow.

LAYER CAKE

METHOD

1. Make the Swiss roll in the usual way; turn it out of the tin and leave to cool on a wire cooling tray, covered with a damp cloth.

2. Cut the Swiss roll *horizontally* into four same-size strips and spread the whole lot with whichever filling, or combination of fillings, you want to use.

3. Roll the first strip up; roll the second strip around the first one, followed by the remaining strips, pressing gently but firmly to seal the edges as you go.

4. Cover the cake with a thick frosting *(see notes, page 204)* to disguise the joins and edges. *N.B. For an even bigger and more impressive cake, make (almost) double the mixture in two Swiss roll tins with the following ingredients:*

8 oz (225 g) plain flour
1 tsp baking powder
8 oz (225 g) butter or margarine
4 eggs
4 tbsp hot water

5. Follow steps 1 – 4 above, rolling up eight strips instead of four.

HONEY, LEMON & YOGHURT CAKE

Like banana cake, carrot cake, ginger cake and fruit muffins, this is the type of thing you find in trendy cafés and leisure centres, where one slice of cake costs more than the whole thing would to make at home. It's really just a basic creamed sponge mixture with ideas above its station, but because it's so fragrant and delicious and has such a lovely soft texture, I think it deserves its place with the other special cakes.

FOR THE CAKE:
6 oz (175 g) plain flour
1 ½ tsp baking powder
6 oz (175 g) butter or margarine
6 oz (175 g) caster sugar
3 eggs (beaten)
4 level tbsp natural yoghurt
1 lemon (juice and zest)
2 tsp honey

FOR THE TOPPING:
1 lemon (juice and zest)
2 oz (50 g) caster sugar

....

1–2 tbsp icing sugar

METHOD
1. Grease and *completely* line an 8″ (21 cm) round cake tin and preheat the oven to Gas Mark 4 (180°C).
2. Cream the butter, sugar, lemon juice and zest in a large mixing bowl until pale and fluffy.
3. Gradually add the beaten eggs a little at a time, taking care not to curdle the mixture.

4. Sift the flour and baking powder into the bowl, followed by the yoghurt and honey and fold it all in together with a metal spoon as quickly as you can without over-beating the mixture.
5. Scoop the mixture into the tin and bake *on one of the lower shelves of the oven* on Gas Mark 4 (180°C) for about one hour.
6. Make the topping when the cake is still warm by mixing the juice and zest of the second lemon in a small saucepan with 2 oz (50 g) sugar and heating for a few minutes until the sugar melts to make a clear syrup. Sprinkle the syrup evenly over the top of the cake and dust with sifted icing sugar. Equally delicious warm or cold.

THE ULTIMATE CHOCOLATE CAKE

Don't use cooking chocolate or any of the bars of chocolate flavoured coating you find in the supermarket's baking section. Regular 'eating' chocolate between 40–60 per cent cocoa solids (look at the list of ingredients on the wrapper) is much better for this cake. It doesn't have to be expensive either; most of the big supermarkets make reasonably good plain chocolate at around 50p for a 4 oz (100 g) bar. For an extra moist sponge, add a couple of tablespoons of natural yoghurt at the same time as the eggs, sugar and melted chocolate – but don't overdo it or you'll end up with a pudding instead of a cake.

6 oz (175 g) self-raising flour
1 tsp baking powder
2 oz cocoa powder
8 oz (225 g) soft brown sugar
8 oz (225 g) butter or margarine
2 heaped tsp instant coffee dissolved in 2 tbsp of boiling water
8 oz (225 g) plain chocolate
3 eggs
2 tbsp golden syrup

OPTIONAL:

2 tbsp natural or Greek yoghurt

METHOD

1. Base-line two 7″ (18 cm) sandwich tins and pre-heat the oven to Gas Mark 4 (180°C).
2. Melt the butter and chocolate (both broken into small pieces) with the dissolved coffee and golden syrup in a heatproof bowl over a pan of boiling water.
3. Meanwhile, sift the flour, baking powder and cocoa powder into a large mixing bowl and make a well in the centre.
4. Add the sugar, beaten eggs and the thick melted chocolate mixture to the well and whisk the whole lot together on maximum speed for about 30 seconds to make a mixture with a smooth, fudgy texture.
5. Divide the mixture equally between the two sandwich tins and bake in the middle (or lower and middle shelves if you can't fit both tins on the same shelf) of the oven for 20 –30 minutes, until the sponges are risen and firm to the touch.
6. Allow to cool slightly while you make the chocolate frosting, then fill and cover the cake and store in an airtight tin. This cake keeps well for at least a week.

TO MAKE THE CHOCOLATE FROSTING:

8 oz (225 g) icing sugar
4 oz (100 g) plain chocolate
1 oz (25 g) butter
1 egg
1 tbsp golden syrup

1. Melt the chocolate, butter and syrup in a bowl over a pan of boiling water.
2. Sift the icing sugar and cocoa powder together into a large mixing bowl and make a well in the centre.
3. Pour the melted chocolate mixture into the well with the egg (or, if the bowl is big enough, add the dry ingredients and the egg to the chocolate mixture) and beat at high speed for about 30 seconds until you've got a thick, smooth icing.
4. Fill and cover the cake, using a flat knife or a fork to make swirls in the icing on the top and sides of the cake.

CHOCOLATE CARAMEL CAKES

FOR THE SHORTBREAD:
6 oz (175 g) butter
4 oz (100 g) caster sugar
12 oz (300 g) plain flour

FOR THE FILLING:
2 x 450 g tins Carnation condensed milk (= 1 pint)
4 oz (100 g) butter
4 tbsp golden syrup

FOR THE TOPPING:
12 oz (300 g) plain chocolate
Small carton of single cream

METHOD

TO MAKE THE SHORTBREAD:

1. Cream the butter and sugar together in a large mixing bowl for no more than a minute. (You're not making a sponge cake so it doesn't have to be especially pale and fluffy.)
2. Add the flour and beat on the lowest speed setting for another minute until the mixture resembles medium-fine breadcrumbs.
3. Press the shortbread mixture into the greased oven tray and bake at Gas Mark 4 (180°C) for about 15 minutes. Don't let the shortbread go brown; it should still be only just golden.

TO MAKE THE FILLING:

4. Put the butter in a large saucepan over a low heat; when it's melted add the condensed milk and the golden syrup and heat gently for a couple of minutes until the ingredients are blended, stirring all the time.
5. Turn the heat up and boil (not too fiercely or you'll get splashed with very hot syrup – and it hurts) for 5–10 minutes, stirring or whisking with a small hand whisk all the time, until you have a light golden brown caramel.
6. Remove from the heat and let the caramel cool slightly for a minute or two, then pour and spread over the shortbread base and leave to cool completely for at least half an hour.

To make the topping:

7. Melt the chocolate in a bowl over a pan of boiling water and stir in the single cream.

8. Pour and spread over the cool caramel and shortbread base with the back of a spoon, making swirling patterns in the chocolate. When the chocolate is starting to set, mark into squares, and when it's cool, cut completely, lifting the chocolate caramel shortbread cakes off the tray with a flat knife and store in an airtight tin.

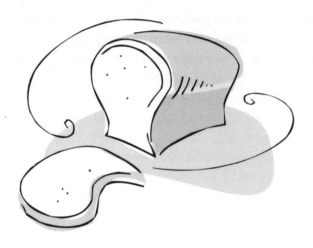

"When you cook it should be an
act of love. To put a frozen bag
in the microwave for your child is
an act of hate."

Raymond Blanc

Not only but also

There's nothing here that you can't buy in the shops ... so why bother? Well, all I can say is, if you can make something better yourself and save money at the same time, it's got to be worth having a go.

Do your bit to help foil the food manufacturers' evil plan to put a morbidly obese child in every classroom; put those oven-ready hash browns back in the freezer, reject that dodgy potato salad, don't eat hot cross buns before Easter, and do try this at home...

QUICK BROWN BREAD

This is perfect for those of us who like the idea of baking our own bread but know we'll never get round to doing it properly. Don't be too heavy handed with the syrup – I've said this in some of the other recipes with golden syrup because, for me, the temptation to ladle it out of the tin in great dollops or squeeze the bottle too hard is overwhelming – otherwise the bread will be too soft and break up easily when you try and cut it. (Turn the loaf upside down when you slice it, in any case. It works better this way for some reason.)

½ lb (225 g) plain wholemeal flour
½ lb (225 g) plain flour
1 tsp salt
1 tsp bicarbonate of soda
1 tsp cream of tartar
¼ pint (125 ml) milk
¼ pint (125 ml) boiling water

1 tbsp golden syrup
1 tsp vinegar

OPTIONAL:
Crushed sunflower seeds, pumpkins seeds, or sesame seeds
sprinkled across the top of the loaf just before it goes into the oven.

METHOD
1. Pre-heat the oven to Gas Mark 5 (190°C) and liberally grease
    a standard 1lb loaf tin.
2. Sift all the dry ingredients into a very large mixing bowl –
    tipping the grains from the wholemeal flour back into the bowl
    afterwards – mix them together and make a well in the centre.
3. Pour ¼ pint (125 ml) of milk into a measuring jug and fill with
    boiling water straight from the kettle to the ¾ pint (375 ml) mark.
4. Add the golden syrup and vinegar to the hot liquid and stir
    for a few seconds to dissolve the syrup.
5. Pour the liquid into the well and mix it all together with a large
    metal spoon to make a loose, sticky dough.
6. Scoop the dough into the loaf tin and use the back of the
    spoon to paddle it down and spread it out as evenly as you
    possibly can. Sprinkle seeds on top if you're using them and
    bake in the middle of the oven, Gas Mark 5 (190°C) for
    30–40 minutes.
7. Turn the loaf out of the tin and tap the bottom; the hollow
    sound it makes means it's done.

SODA BREAD

This isn't the best bread for toast and sandwiches, but on its own
with butter, or as something to have with soups and stews, it's great.
(It also keeps for a couple of days wrapped in foil and freezes well.)

If you want to add any of the herbs or seeds listed below, mix them in with the dry ingredients at the beginning and keep a bit back to scatter across the top just before the loaf goes into the oven.

DRY INGREDIENTS:
12 oz (300 g) self-raising wholemeal flour
4 oz (100 g) self-raising white flour
1 oz (25 g) brown sugar
1 tsp salt
2 tsp bicarbonate of soda

...

1 oz (25 g) butter
¼ pint (125 ml) milk
About half a large (500 g) pot of natural yoghurt
2 oz (50 g) porridge oats

OPTIONAL:
2 tsp dried (or 2 sprigs of fresh) rosemary, thyme, or sage
2 tbsp seeds (pumpkin, sunflower, caraway) roughly chopped

METHOD
1. Pre-heat the oven to Gas Mark 4 (180°C) and grease a standard baking tray.
2. Mix the dry ingredients together in a large bowl; add the butter in small pieces and rub in, then make a well in the centre.
3. Mix the milk and yoghurt together and pour most of the liquid into the centre, keeping a couple of tablespoonfuls back for brushing over the top of the finished loaf.
4. Mix the liquid in quickly using your hands to make a soft (but not too sticky) dough, then turn the dough out onto a floured surface. Knead it very lightly for a minute and form into a round cottage-style loaf.

5. Place the loaf on the greased tray and cut a deep cross on the top; brush the remains of the milk/yoghurt mixture all over the surface (you can use your hands if you don't have a pastry brush) and sprinkle over the porridge oats, or whatever other herbs or seeds you want to use, if any.

6. Bake in the oven for 30–40 minutes and allow the loaf to cool for half an hour before eating.

GARLIC BREAD

Garlic bread works best with baguettes, but there's nothing to stop you warming up any other type of bread at the bottom of the oven, wrapped in foil, then spreading it with garlic butter after a few minutes, once the bread's hot enough to melt the butter.

4 oz (100 g) butter
2 garlic cloves, crushed
¼ tsp salt
1 baguette

OPTIONAL:
2 tsp parsley
Black pepper

METHOD

1. Take the butter out of the fridge for a few minutes first to soften it up, crush the garlic and beat the ingredients together.

2. Make one long cut along the length of the baguette underneath and spread the loaf liberally with the garlic butter on both sides.

3. Turn the loaf up the right way and make deep, regular cuts all the way across the top, about halfway down to the bottom.

4. Wrap the loaf in foil and warm in the bottom of a hot oven, Gas Mark 6 (200°C) for about 15–20 minutes, taking the foil off 5 minutes before the end for a crunchier crust.

PATES

These are two of the simplest recipes for pate you'll find anywhere as there's very little preparation or cooking involved. They both work well as a starter or snack, especially with vegetable sticks and French bread or a bowl of tortilla chips on the side. The chicken liver pate is also nice on hot toast with lots of mustard.

CHICKEN LIVER PATE

½ lb (225 g) chicken livers
1 onion
2 cloves of garlic
2 tsp thyme
2 tbsp butter
½ small glass of sherry or brandy
2 tbsp single cream

METHOD
1. Clean and cut the livers into small pieces, removing any skin or fatty bits, then peel and finely chop the onion and crush the garlic.
2. Melt 1 tbsp butter in a large saucepan, add the liver, onion, garlic and thyme, and fry for about 5 minutes, then turn the heat down, cover with a lid and cook gently for another 5 minutes.
3. Transfer everything to a large mixing bowl with a slotted spoon in order to leave most of the liquid behind in the pan.
4. Blend on the lowest speed setting for a minute, adding a fresh bit of butter (about 1 tbsp) with the sherry and cream and

then blend for a few seconds more.

5. Put the pate into a small casserole dish and chill in the fridge for about an hour. Eat within four days.

KIPPER PATE

You can use pre-packed boil-in-the-bag kippers for this, which means the skin and most of the bones will already have been removed.

$^{1}/_{2}$ lb (225 g) kippers
300 g tub low fat cream cheese
1 lemon (juice)
1 clove of garlic
Black pepper

METHOD

1. Follow the instructions on the packet for boil-in-the-bag kippers, or grill or fry them gently with a little lump of butter for about 10 minutes.
2. Flake the kippers, double-checking for large bones, then put the fish in a large mixing bowl with the cream cheese, garlic, lemon juice and black pepper.
3. Either beat everything together with a wooden spoon, or use an electric whisk to get a fairly smooth, creamy paste in a matter of seconds. Cover with a lid and chill the pate in the fridge for about an hour. Use within four days.

GUACAMOLE

2 large avocados
1 or 2 tbsp from a tin of chopped tomatoes
$^{1}/_{2}$ tsp chilli powder or cayenne pepper

1 clove of garlic, crushed
1 tbsp natural yoghurt
Lime juice to taste (say 2 tsp)

METHOD

1. Mash the avocados in a bowl, add the rest of the ingredients, mix well, cover with a layer of clingfilm and keep refrigerated for up to 2 days.

HUMMUS

14 oz (410 g) tin of chick peas
4 oz (100 g) sesame seeds
2 tbsp olive oil
2 cloves of garlic
3 big tbsp natural yoghurt
Juice of 2 lemons (or 4–6 tbsp lemon juice, according to taste)
Salt & pepper

METHOD

1. Put the sesame seeds and olive oil in a blender or food processor and whiz for about a minute, scraping everything away from the sides once or twice if you need to.
2. Drain the tin of chick peas and add them to the blender with the rest of the ingredients, in no particular order, and blend on high speed for a couple of minutes.
3. Adjust seasoning and chill in the fridge for a couple of hours before eating. Keeps for about a week.

ROASTED NUTS

A great alternative to heavily salted and (smelly) dry-roasted peanuts.

Large bags of unsalted nuts can be found in local Asian shops and the international section of most major supermarkets. If they haven't already been shelled and peeled you can blanch them at home by soaking them in a bowl of boiling water for a few minutes, then straining through a colander and plunging them into cold water, so the skins slide off easily.

For 1 lb (500 g) of nuts – cashews, peanuts, almonds or hazelnuts – use 1 ½ oz (37 g) of butter, 1 teaspoon of salt and any one of the following three seasonings:

1 tbsp curry powder

1 tbsp paprika

1 tsp chilli powder + 2 tsp of cumin

METHOD
1. Pre-heat the oven to Gas Mark 2 (150°C).
2. Melt the butter on a roasting tray or large ovenproof dish, mix well with the spices, then add the nuts and give the tray a good shake, making sure all the nuts are basted in the seasoned butter.
3. Roast in a cool oven for about 30 minutes, allow to cool and store in an airtight tin.

MAYONNAISE

Making mayonnaise is such a doddle, it's worth doing at home at least some of the time (especially in the summer when you're eating lots of salads), so when some beady-eyed domestic diva asks if you made it yourself you can truthfully say 'yes'. (Ha!)

(Although you're supposed to use powdered mustard I always buy readymade and use it straight from the jar, and it's fine.)

3 egg yolks
$\frac{1}{2}$ pint (250 ml) olive oil
3–4 tbsp cider vinegar
2 tbsp lemon juice
$\frac{1}{2}$ tsp English mustard
Salt & white pepper

METHOD
1. Separate the eggs and put the yolks in a cold bowl with the mustard, salt and white pepper; mix the vinegar and lemon juice together in a cup.
2. Beat the egg yolks for a minute, then start adding the oil, drop by drop to prevent the eggs curdling. Once the mayonnaise starts to thicken the oil can be added in a steady stream – but don't stop beating. (As always, it's better to use an electric hand whisk.)
3. Add half the vinegar and lemon juice as soon as the mayonnaise starts getting too thick to work with; then carry on adding the rest of the oil.
4. Beat the rest of the vinegar and lemon juice in – the mayonnaise should be thick and smooth – and adjust the seasoning, adding more vinegar if you like a runnier texture (although this makes it salad cream rather than mayonnaise).

POTATO SALAD

Use about half the quantity of mayonnaise made from the above recipe for this amount of potatoes, mixed with a couple of tablespoons of natural yoghurt.

SERVES 6–12:
2 lbs (1 kg) potatoes
3 spring onions
Mayonnaise
Natural yoghurt
Chives
Parsley
Lemon juice
Salt & pepper

METHOD
1. Wash and boil the potatoes in their skins until just soft, then leave to cool for a few minutes. (Either remove the skins while the potatoes are still warm, or leave them on.)
2. Dice the potatoes and add to a large bowl with the mayonnaise, yoghurt, chopped spring onions, herbs, salt & pepper; mix gently and adjust the seasoning and consistency according to taste.

HASH BROWNS

Hash browns are high in fat wherever they come from, although homemade ones less so, and they also contain more of the healthier ingredients per portion.

It goes without saying that they taste better too. (Add a few chives or some parsley to the raw mixture to prove you didn't get them out of a packet.)

THIS IS ENOUGH FOR ABOUT 16 GOOD-SIZE HASH BROWNS:
2 lb (1 kg) potatoes
1 onion
3 tbsp butter, melted
3 tbsp plain, or plain wholemeal flour

METHOD

1. Peel and grate the potatoes, then wash well in a colander to rinse the starch away and squeeze dry in an old, clean tea towel.
2. Grate the onion and mix with the grated potatoes in a large bowl.
3. Sift the flour into the bowl, add the melted butter and mix the whole lot together.
4. Make the mixture into cakes with your hands and shallow fry in very hot oil for a few minutes on each side, flattening them out a bit with the vegetable slice.

TO FREEZE:

1. If you want to freeze hash browns, cook them first, drain on kitchen roll and allow to cool, then layer with greaseproof paper, place in a large food bag and freeze.
2. Re-heat straight from the freezer by placing the hash browns on an ovenproof tray and cooking on Gas Mark 7 (220°C) for 15–20 minutes.

HOT CROSS BUNS

Hot cross buns are nowhere as special as they used to be when you could only buy them on Good Friday, but as they're easy enough to do at home I think it's worth making them once, or even twice a year. There's no time to put your feet up; you need to move straight from one stage to the next, but having said that, the whole process is very straightforward and only takes about an hour from start to finish.

I made hot cross buns for the first time last Easter after my son made them at school and gave me a rough idea of the recipe at home. Although they weren't much like the shop-bought variety they were still good – but I don't know how his buns turned out because he didn't save one for me...

Makes about 12 hot cross buns (or 18 minis):
1lb (450 g) strong plain flour – or strong wholemeal flour
1 sachet dried yeast
4 oz (100 g) sultanas
½ tsp mixed spice
½ tsp cinnamon
½ tsp nutmeg
4 oz (100 g) butter or margarine
1 egg, (beaten)
½ pint (125 ml) milk and water (about half and half)
4 oz (100 g) sugar (caster or soft brown)

For the crosses:
4 oz (100 g) strong white flour
2 oz (50 g) butter or margarine
1–2 tbsp water

To glaze:
4 tbsp sugar
4 tbsp water

N.B. You need to prove the dough in a warm place – the airing cupboard is ideal – in which case you can wrap the dough in clingfilm. Otherwise, use your oven on the lowest possible setting, putting the dough on a greased oven tray – the one you're going to use for baking the buns will do – and covering with a clean, damp tea towel.

Method

1. Gently heat the milk and water in a saucepan (don't let it boil) and once it's warm, stir in the sugar, then sprinkle the dried yeast on top and leave to stand for about 10 minutes while you wash the sultanas in warm water. (Dry the sultanas in an old, clean tea towel.)

2. Sift the flour and spices into a large mixing bowl and rub in the butter until the mixture resembles medium-fine breadcrumbs.
3. Make a well in the centre, add the beaten egg and warm milk and mix everything together with a fork to make a firm dough.
4. Turn the dough out onto a floured surface and knead for about 5 minutes, then leave to prove for about 10 minutes (*see above*).
5. Place the dough on a floured surface and knead again for a couple of minutes, then shape into rolls – about the size of a satsuma – flatten them slightly and place on the greased baking sheet. (You might want to use 2 baking sheets so you can spread the buns out a bit more.)
6. Lightly make a cross on top of each bun with the side of a knife and prove for a further 10 minutes.

MAKING THE CROSSES:
7. While the buns are proving, rub in the butter and flour and mix to a firm dough with the water, then turn the dough onto a floured surface; roll it out as thinly as you can without breaking and mark it into long, thin strips with a sharp knife.
8. Dunk the strips into a mug of cold milk and water and stick them to the buns where you marked out the crosses, then using your fingers or a pastry brush, lightly glaze all the buns with the milk and water.
9. Bake in the oven, Gas Mark 4 (180°C) for about 20 minutes, until the buns are a light, golden brown.

MAKING THE GLAZE:
10. While the buns are in the oven, heat the water and sugar in a deep-sided saucepan until the sugar is dissolved, then allow to boil for a few minutes to make a fairly thin syrup.
11. Take the buns from the oven and while they're still warm, brush them with the syrup and leave to cool.

HONEYCOMB

Use a very large aluminium saucepan and don't worry about the shocking state of the pan afterwards; it only needs a five-minute soak in very hot water and, hey presto, it's clean again.

8 heaped tbsp sugar
8 heaped tbsp golden syrup
4 tbsp water
4 rounded tsp bicarbonate of soda

METHOD
1. Lightly oil a sheet of greaseproof paper and put it in a shallow bowl, plate or cake tin.
2. Put the sugar, golden syrup and water in a large saucepan over a moderate heat, mix it all together and stir continuously with a wooden spoon.
3. Let the syrup boil for up to 5 minutes – keep your eye on the clock – by which time it should be a rich, golden brown (but not too dark, you don't want it burnt).
4. Quickly add the bicarbonate of soda, still stirring rapidly, and get the pan off the heat as the honeycomb froths and rises up the pan.
5. Scrape the honeycomb onto the greaseproof paper immediately and leave to set for about an hour before breaking it up into chunks.

GINGER BEER

I first made ginger beer in primary school with the same teacher who taught us to make miniature pancakes on top of an old baked bean tin with a candle underneath... (Mrs Jones, where are you now? And can you imagine what the health & safety brigade would say about candles in the classroom today?)

Anyway, I remember being bitterly disappointed after all the waiting, never having tried ginger beer before, and thinking it tasted revolting. Now I like it, and this process is so straightforward it's a good project for kids to have a go at during those long school holidays – or you can start on a Saturday and finish it off the following weekend.

Like other beer and ciders, ginger beer can also be used in cooking *(see Ginger Beer Pork and Honey & Ginger Glazed Carrots in Chapter 3: Make Dinner, Not Excuses)*.

METHOD
TO START:
½ pint (125 ml) fresh, cold water
1 tbsp ground ginger
1 heaped tsp soft brown sugar

1. Put the cold water, ginger and sugar in a clean, dry jar with a tight-fitting lid, and give it a good shake.
2. Every day for the next 7 DAYS add 1 heaped teaspoon of ginger and 1 level teaspoon of sugar to the jar; then holding the jar by the lid, gently swish round for a few seconds before leaving it to stand.

TO MAKE THE GINGER BEER (LEAVE FOR AT LEAST 12 HOURS AFTER THE FINAL ADDITION OF SUGAR AND GINGER):
2 x 2 litre bottles of still water
2 lemons
1 ½ mugs of soft brown sugar
3 mugs of boiling water
1 level teaspoon of dried yeast

N.B. To make an alcoholic version, add a double measure of whisky (2 x 35 ml) – or a miniature – to a 2 litre bottle of ginger beer at the final stage.

1. Fill (or half fill) the kettle with water from one of the 2 litre bottles of mineral water.
2. Using an old, clean tea towel, carefully strain the ginger and sugar mixture from the jar through the cloth, into a very large mixing bowl. If the tea towel is very old and threadbare, fold it in half so as not to let too much of the sediment through.
3. Squeeze both lemons through a clean part of the cloth – squeezing the cloth gently with your fingers to let as much juice into the bowl as you can.
4. Pour three mugs of boiling water into the bowl and add the yeast and sugar, stirring for a couple of minutes until all the sugar has dissolved.
5. Allow the liquid to stand for half an hour, then strain through another old, clean tea towel (or thoroughly rinse the first one and use it again; doesn't matter if it's damp) and add the entire contents of the second 2 litre bottle of water, plus whatever remains from the first bottle, and mix well.
6. Use a jug or funnel to pour the ginger beer into the two 2 litre bottles (adding the whisky if you're using it) and refrigerate. As soon as the ginger beer is chilled, it's ready to drink. *(If you find there's still a lot of sediment in the bottle after 24 hours, strain the ginger beer through an old, clean tea towel again, rinse out the bottle and pour the drink back in.)*

TOFFEE APPLES

The amounts given here are enough for eight toffee apples but it's a good idea to make a greater quantity of toffee than you need so you've got more to play around with; the syrup thickens very rapidly as it cools, which makes it trickier to get a nice, even layer of toffee over the last few apples.

MAKES 8 TOFFEE APPLES:
12 oz soft brown or caster sugar
2 oz (50 g) butter
4 oz (100 g) golden syrup
1 tsp lemon juice
¼ pint (125 ml) water

METHOD
1. Lightly grease a large sheet of greaseproof paper and have a large bowl of cold water ready beside the stove.
2. Wash apples in lukewarm water and dry thoroughly, then push a lolly stick into each one, where the stalk used to be, about halfway through.
3. Put all the ingredients into a large saucepan and stir over a low heat for a few minutes until the sugar has completely dissolved.
4. Increase the heat to medium-high and allow the syrup to boil fairly rapidly for about 15 minutes, stirring occasionally.
5. After 20 minutes (not a minute more with this quantity) drop about half a teaspoon of the boiling syrup into the cold water; if it hardens immediately it's ready. A fudgier sort of toffee means it needs to be boiled a little longer – coat the apples with too-soft toffee and you'll never get it off your teeth.
6. TEST AGAIN AFTER ONE MINUTE.
7. When the toffee is ready, take the pan off the heat and tilt it slightly, making it easier to dip the apples.
8. Swirl the apples around in the syrup one at a time, as quickly as you can, then plunge them straight into the cold water and leave them upside down on the greaseproof paper to dry completely.

BOTTLING IT

For chutney, fruit spread and grapefruit curd (see below) the jars always need to be warm – regardless of whether the produce is going in hot or cold – in order to prevent mildew forming. You can warm the jars by rinsing in very hot water and drying them quickly, but an easier way is to put the jars in the microwave; about 45 seconds (or 1 minute) on high should do it.

CHUTNEY

This is great as a dip, or with cheese, jacket potatoes and cold meats, or try adding a couple of spoonfuls to curry, pasta sauce and nut roasts for extra flavour.

You should get about six standard size jam jars out of this lot, so if you want to make less, halve the quantities.

5–6 large cooking apples (i.e. Bramleys)
1 head of celery
2 onions
1lb sultanas
1 pint (500 ml) brown (or white) malt vinegar
½ pint (250 ml) water
12 oz (350 g) Demerara sugar
1 level tbsp salt
1 heaped tsp mixed spice

METHOD
1. Wash the sultanas in warm water.
2. Top and tail the celery and remove the leaves, peel the onions, then roughly chop the vegetables into small chunks. (Leave the apples till the end to stop them going brown.)

3. Pour the vinegar and water into a large saucepan and add the prepared vegetables, sultanas, salt, sugar and spice.
4. Cut the apples into quarters (or even smaller), peel, core, cut into small chunks and add to the pan.
5. Give everything a good stir and bring to the boil over a moderate heat, then turn the heat right down and simmer very gently for 1 ½– 2 hours, stirring occasionally.
6. When the chutney looks ready, i.e. thick, pulpy and sweet smelling, pour it into a large bowl, cover with an old, clean tea towel and leave to stand for at least a few hours, and preferably overnight.
7. Bottle in warm, dry jars *(see above)* and store in the cupboard.

SOFT FRUIT SPREAD

Jam making for absolute beginners; this is as easy as it gets, but because it doesn't keep quite as well as regular jam, which is made with twice the amount of sugar, store it in the fridge and use within a couple of weeks once the jar is opened.

Any soft fruit, or a mixture of soft fruits will do, i.e. raspberries, blackberries, blackcurrants, redcurrants and cherries. If you get the chance to pick blackberries for free at the end of August/beginning of September, make the most of it; they freeze well and you can do lots with them.

You should get a couple of jars from this amount of fruit and sugar, so increase the quantities and use a larger pan if you want to make more.

2 lbs (1 kg) soft fruit
1lb (450 g) granulated sugar
2 lemons

METHOD

1. Put the fruit in a saucepan with the sugar, juice from both lemons and a little water – unless the fruit is already very wet and running with juice, in which case you may not need any – *and heat very gently for a few minutes*, stirring often with a wooden spoon, to give the sugar time to dissolve.

2. Turn the heat up and boil fairly rapidly for 20–30 minutes until the jam thickens and gels and you can separate it in the saucepan for a couple of seconds when you run the wooden spoon through the middle.

3. Remove the jam from the heat and let it stand for about 10 minutes, then pour it into warm, dry jars.

4. Leave to cool for another 10 minutes, then cover.

GRAPEFRUIT CURD

Homemade fruit curd is similar to shop-bought, but less solid, with a purer taste and texture. If you'd rather have a thicker, jelly-like curd, add a teaspoon of cornflour mixed with a tablespoonful of water and a few drops of lemon juice at the end; thick or thin, it's equally good on bread and crackers or as a filling in cakes and pastries. To make lemon curd, just use 2 lemons (rind and juice) instead of one grapefruit.

MAKES ROUGHLY ONE STANDARD SIZE JAM JAR:
1 grapefruit – grated rind and juice
8 oz (225 g) caster sugar
3 oz (75 g) butter
3 eggs

METHOD

1. Melt the butter in a saucepan over a moderate heat.
2. Add the sugar with the finely grated rind and juice of the grapefruit and stir for a couple of minutes until all the sugar has dissolved.
3. Pour in the beaten egg and stir briskly and continuously with a wooden spoon to prevent the egg separating while the mixture thickens. (Don't panic if any little white flecks of egg do develop; you can get rid of these when you strain the curd at the end.)
4. After about 10 minutes the curd should have reached the consistency of custard, which means it's ready.
5. Strain through a sieve into a measuring jug and pour straight into the warm jar. Leave to cool for about 30 minutes, then put the lid on and store it in the fridge.

FIGGY PUDDING

I've always liked the idea of Christmas pudding made with figs (as the song suggests) but by far the best thing about this pudding – apart from the short list of ingredients – is the fact that it doesn't need time to mature, meaning you can make it a couple of days before Christmas when you're feeling Christmassy, rather than in October when you can't bear the thought of winter, let alone 'Winterval' (as it will never be known in my house).

The quantities here make three 1 lb puddings, so if you only want one large pudding to get you and your family through Christmas and Boxing Day, halve all the measurements except for the sherry and make one big pudding in a 1 ½ –2 lb pudding basin, in which case you should steam it for the maximum four hours.

Cover each pudding with a double thickness of greaseproof paper with a pleat in the middle to allow for any expansion, then put a layer of foil over the top of the greaseproof, also with a pleat in the middle, and fold the foil tightly around the rim, or secure with string.

Finally, if you want to put a coin in for good luck (£1 must be the going rate these days), wrap it in foil and pop it in before covering the pudding for the first time.

FOR 3 X 1 LB PUDDINGS:
1 lb (400–500 g) fresh white breadcrumbs
2 oz (50 g) self-raising flour
4 oz (100 g) soft brown sugar
4 oz (100 g) suet
1 lb dried figs
1 lb mixed fruit
3 tsp mixed spice
½ tsp salt
1 oz (25 g) flaked almonds
¼ pint (125 ml) sherry or brandy
3 fl oz (90 ml) milk
2 eggs, beaten

METHOD
1. Grease the pudding basins with butter.
2. Mix the breadcrumbs with the sifted flour, suet, sugar, salt and spices in a very large mixing bowl.
3. Wash the mixed fruit in warm water, dry thoroughly in an old, clean tea towel and chop the figs into small pieces (wash them too, unless the packaging states 'ready to eat').
4. Crumble up the flaked almonds with your hands and add them to the bowl with the fruit, followed by the sherry, milk and beaten eggs.
5. Stir thoroughly for a minute, making sure everything is

combined, then put the mixture into the prepared pudding basins, cover and leave to stand overnight.

6. Steam the puddings for 3–4 hours (depending on size) in a saucepan of boiling water, topping up the level of water every now and then to prevent the saucepan from boiling dry.
7. After steaming, allow the puddings to cool for at least 1 hour before removing the foil and greaseproof paper and covering with fresh foil and greaseproof paper.
8. Store puddings at room temperature and steam again for a further 2 hours before serving with brandy butter, custard or cream.

BRANDY BUTTER

There's no reason why you can't make brandy butter with sherry instead of brandy or, as my dad often did, with whisky.

3 oz (75 g) unsalted butter
3 oz (75 g) icing sugar
2 tbsp spirit

METHOD

1. Keep the butter at room temperature, then beat it in a mixing bowl with an electric hand whisk until it's light and fluffy – or use a wooden spoon, if you've got enough strength left in your arm (it's Christmas remember).
2. Gradually beat in the icing sugar, followed by the brandy or other spirit, and chill in the fridge for an hour before serving.

FUDGE

There's something upmarket and slightly sophisticated about fudge compared with your average chewy toffee, but although it gives the impression that it's been made with great skill by someone who really knows their stuff, all you need to do is spend a few minutes stirring butter, sugar and milk together while you think about something more important. Just like the Honey, Lemon & Yoghurt Cake in Chapter 8, any kind of homemade fudge – chocolate, coffee, fruity, extra creamy, coconut – not only looks good, it has the magical effect of making the person who made it look good too. Result!

The quantities given here make 36 good-size cubes in an 8″ (21 cm) square cake tin, or similar, but if you haven't made fudge before and are a bit unsure, you may want to make only half this amount, in which case you shouldn't need to boil the mixture for any longer than 15 minutes (start testing after 10 minutes).

Once you've taken the fudge off the heat it's better to cool it down quickly rather than beating it by hand for at least another 10 minutes while you stand around wondering if it's going to work, so stand the pan in a shallow bowl of cold water (the washing up bowl will do) or, if you can bear to get another pan dirty, scrape the fudge into a clean, cool one. After a couple of minutes the fudge will start to thicken and lose its shine, becoming dull and slightly grainy – exactly how you'd expect fudge to look – then all you have to do is add the flavouring and get it in the tin.

MAKES 36 CUBES:
2 lb (1 kg) sugar
6 oz (175 g) unsalted butter
1 tin (410 g) of evaporated milk
Roughly ¼ pint (125 ml) milk

METHOD
1. Melt the butter in a large saucepan while you lightly grease and long-strip-line a square or rectangular cake tin.
2. Pour the tin of evaporated milk into a measuring jug then top up to the 1 pint (500 ml) mark with the milk.

3. Add the milk and sugar to the pan over a low heat and leave it for about 5 minutes, stirring occasionally, until the sugar has dissolved.

4. Bring to the boil, then boil rapidly for 15–20 minutes, stirring continuously, until the syrup reaches the 'soft ball stage', meaning ½ teaspoon of syrup dropped into a cup of cold water holds its shape and looks and feels like a piece of soft toffee when you squeeze it.

5. Remove the pan from the heat and allow the fudge to cool for a few minutes *(see above)*, beating almost constantly, then add the flavouring and scrape it into the   prepared tin.

6. Mark the fudge into squares after about 15 minutes; leave it in the tin for at least 2 hours to cool completely, then lift it out, cut it up and store in an airtight tin.

COFFEE & VANILLA FUDGE:
1 tsp instant coffee dissolved in 1 tbsp boiling water
2 tsp vanilla extract

1. While the fudge is cooling, quickly dissolve 1 tsp of instant coffee in a cup with 1 tbsp of boiling water, then mix with the vanilla extract and thoroughly beat the liquid into the fudge.

CHOCOLATE MARBLE FUDGE:
3 oz (75 g) plain chocolate

1. Break the chocolate into pieces and melt in a bowl over a saucepan of boiling water while you make the fudge.

2. As soon as the fudge is cool and ready to go into the tin, pour the chocolate into the middle of the fudge and stir *only once or twice* in clean, sweeping movements, to create a marbled effect. Pour the fudge into the tin and leave to set.

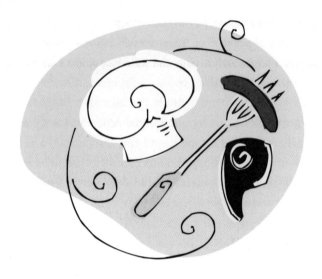

"The most remarkable thing about my
mother is that for thirty years she served
the family nothing but leftovers.
The original meal has never been found."

Calvin Trillin

Weekly menu planning

It's not only desperate housewives who plan a week's-worth of evening meals in advance, so don't be put off if you haven't tried this before. Go shopping with a list and you're far less likely to waste time wandering up and down the aisles, absent-mindedly loading up your trolley with random items.

Is there anyone who's never gone to the supermarket for a loaf of bread and come out half an hour later with three carrier bags bulging with impulse buys? I read recently that in Britain we waste a staggering, and scarcely believable, £23 billion a year on food, much of which gets chucked away while it's still perfectly edible (whatever the sell-by date says), mainly because we buy whatever takes our fancy at the time without thinking about when and how we're going to use it.

Such is the seductive power of the supermarket, and if, like me, you struggle with portion control – meaning your dinners for four people could easily feed six – a menu plan should help you get your worst excesses under control. The other thing I like about planning meals in advance is, contrary to what you might expect, it completely takes the focus away from food. Once you've worked out the menu for the week and done the shopping you can just forget all about it.

If lack of inspiration is your biggest problem – apparently the average British household recycles the same six or seven meals from one week to the next – you'll find a few minutes of planning means you can go for weeks without eating the same thing twice.

Another benefit is the rollover effect; make twice as much as you need of some things for the same amount of effort, then use what's left over to make a completely hassle-free meal the next day.

Best of all, not only does a plan save time, it can also save you a lot of money. The food for the menus in this chapter was bought in five of our major supermarkets, and although the price and quality of some items varies considerably, as the costing shows, it's possible to spend as little as £25 on family dinners for one working week.

These menu plans only cater for Monday to Friday, but you'll probably find you have enough food left at the weekend for at least one more meal, so I think it's fair to say they give a pretty good indication of how economical you can be if you put your mind to it. Of course, you also need to buy washing powder and toothpaste, not to mention food for breakfast, lunch and snacks, but most household items last longer than a week, as do large bags of pasta, rice, flour, sugar, porridge oats, nuts and seeds; also herbs, spices, eggs, stock cubes, oils, gravy granules, tomato puree, honey, jam, lemon and lime juice, vinegar and pickles, so often it's only the freshest ingredients you need to buy on a weekly basis.

Still on the subject of saving money, I'd rather buy own-brand toiletries and the cheapest crisps, biscuits, bin liners, washing up liquid and so on, and spend more money where it matters, on good quality meat, organic milk, fresh vegetables, free-range chicken and eggs. All supermarkets often arrange and market special offers to get shoppers hooked on things before they put the prices up, but it's up to you to make this strategy work in your favour by taking advantage of a good buy, then moving on as soon as something becomes too expensive. I love avocados, but when they go from 37p each to 65p then 75p in the space of a week, as they did recently, I can live without them for a while, just as I can live without apples when I can't find any English ones amongst a sea of fruit from Argentina to Zambia and everywhere else except Britain. Never forget how much choice you have, and how many rival supermarkets there are out there competing for your custom.

Even if you don't have to stick to a budget there's something very liberating about saving money in the supermarket. In fact, it's hard not to feel a little bit smug sometimes, so just give yourself a pat on the back – and see if you can't convince all the less disciplined shoppers you know to see the error of their ways.

THE MENUS

WEEK 1	TESCO	£24.06
Monday:	Chilli Con Carne & Rice	
Tuesday:	Chilli & Chips	
Wednesday:	Veggie Burgers & Potato Wedges	
Thursday:	Chinese Chicken Stir Fry	
Friday:	Frankfurters & DIY Pasta Sauce	

WEEK 2	ASDA	£24.62
Monday:	Roast Chicken	
Tuesday:	Chicken & Leek Casserole	
Wednesday:	Bubble, Bangers & Beans	
Thursday:	Kedgeree	
Friday:	Cheese & Spinach Omelette	

WEEK 3	SAINSBURY'S	£20.66
Monday:	Boiled Bacon & Roasted Vegetables	
Tuesday:	Vegetable Tortilla	
Wednesday:	Pork Meatballs, Tagliatelle & Tomato Sauce	
Thursday:	Stuffed Peppers	
Friday:	Pacific Pie	

WEEK 4	MORRISONS	£24.17
Monday:	Liver, Bacon & Onions	
Tuesday:	Tomato & Red Lentil Soup	
Wednesday:	Salmon & Tomato Pasta Bake	
Thursday:	Pork Ribs, Sausages & Rice	
Friday:	Bread Roll Pizzas	

WEEK 5	WAITROSE	£39.43
Monday:	Corned Beef Hash	
Tuesday:	Fish Finger Pie	
Wednesday:	Spaghetti Bolognese	
Thursday:	Curried Nut Roast	
Friday:	Gammon Steaks, Egg & Homemade Chips	

WEEK ONE

MONDAY:	Chilli Con Carne
TUESDAY:	Chilli and Chips
WEDNESDAY:	Veggie Burgers & Potato Wedges
THURSDAY:	Chinese Chicken Stir Fry
FRIDAY:	Frankfurters & DIY Pasta Sauce

THE SHOPPING LIST

Lean steak mince	£2.72
Free-range chicken portions	£4.47
Frankfurters	0.98
Kidney beans	0.15
Chick peas	0.40
Mozzarella cheese	0.98
Pasta quills	0.19
Long grain rice	0.49

Mushrooms	£1.15
Chinese Stir fry vegetables	£1.28
Potatoes	£1.58
Avocados (4 @ 37p)	£1.48
Spinach	£1.29
Tomatoes	0.98
Carrots	0.35
Broccoli	0.52
Onions	0.28
Courgettes	£1.33
Peppers – mixed	£1.48
Noodles	£1.07
Porridge Oats	0.41
Wholemeal flour	0.79
Tomato puree	0.48
Eggs (12 free-range)	£1.39
Tortilla chips	0.55
	£24.06

WEEK ONE: THE RECIPES

MONDAY:
CHILLI CON CARNE & RICE: *(see Chapter 3: Make Dinner, Not Excuses)*.

TUESDAY:
CHILLI & CHIPS
I always buy the cheapest supermarket own-brand plain tortilla chips (when I can get them; they sell out so quickly), not only because they're irresistible at less than 20p for a large bag, they

contain less salt and are completely free from artificial colouring and flavourings, none of which you need anyway when you've got chilli.

Remains of yesterday's Chilli
1 or 2 bags of tortilla chips
Grated mozzarella cheese
Avocado
Tomatoes (at least one per person)

METHOD
1. Re-heat the Chilli on Gas Mark 4 (180°C) in a large ovenproof dish covered with foil (or a lid) for about 20 minutes until the food is piping hot. Alternatively, cover with a lid and re-heat in the microwave on high for about 5 minutes, taking the Chilli out and giving it a good stir halfway through.
2. Empty a packet of tortilla chips over the chilli, mix them up a bit with the meaty sauce, then sprinkle liberally with grated cheese and return to the oven, or flash under the grill for a couple of minutes, so the cheese melts and the edges of the tortilla chips on the top brown ever so slightly. (Don't let them burn.)
3. Serve with chunks of avocado and tomato wedges.

WEDNESDAY:
VEGGIE BURGERS & POTATO WEDGES: (*for Veggie Burgers see Chapter 3: Make Dinner, Not Excuses*).
Approximately 3–4 small potatoes per person

TO MAKE THE POTATO WEDGES:
1. Wash the potatoes with a nailbrush in a bowl of cold water and cut each one into sixths or eighths, depending on size.
1. Pre-heat the oil or whatever fat you're using in a large ovenproof dish (as if you were going to roast potatoes), pop

the wedges in, sprinkle with paprika, baste with the hot oil and bake for about 30 minutes until they're as brown and crisp as you like them, basting them again with the peppery oil about halfway through the cooking time.

2. Serve with sweetcorn and something green; French beans, curly kale or broccoli, for example.

THURSDAY:
CHINESE CHICKEN STIR FRY

This is more or less the same as the Quorn Stir Fry in Chapter 4: Quick Fixes, except you'll need to make sure the meat's cooked through before you add the stir fry vegetables and noodles. (First rinse the pan out with a little boiling water with the chicken inside, then strain the liquid off and add clean oil. I don't know what Gordon Ramsay would make of this, but it works for me so don't worry too much. He'll never know.)

FRIDAY:
FRANKFURTERS & DIY PASTA SAUCE

This is just a variation of the recipe for DIY Pasta Sauce in Chapter 3: Make Dinner, Not Excuses. (There can't be much nutritional value in a frankfurter, but does it really matter when they taste this good and you've got all the vegetables you need in the pasta sauce?)

WEEK TWO

MONDAY:	Roast Chicken
TUESDAY:	Chicken & Leek Casserole
WEDNESDAY:	Bubble, Bangers & Beans
THURSDAY:	Kedgeree
FRIDAY:	Cheese & Spinach Omelette

THE SHOPPING LIST:

1 free-range chicken	£4.83
18 sausages (82% pork)	£5.00
Smoked Mackerel	£1.49
Cheese	£1.75
Eggs (12 free-range)	£1.75
Milk	£1.40
1 can condensed chicken soup	0.48
Brown rice	0.60
Baked beans	0.17
Plum tomatoes	0.13
Oven chips	0.44
Potatoes	£1.24
Frozen peas	0.99
Carrots	0.68
Spinach	£1.58
Leeks	0.68
Broccoli	0.58
Parsnips	0.52
White cabbage	0.39
	£24.62

WEEK TWO: THE RECIPES

MONDAY:

ROAST CHICKEN WITH ROAST POTATOES AND PARSNIPS, WHITE CABBAGE, CARROTS AND PEAS.

With plenty of vegetables, one large chicken should be enough to make a meal for four people two nights' running, so try not to scoff the whole lot in one sitting.

If, on the other hand, you're truly worthy of domestic goddess status, you'll use the leftovers to make stock for Chicken Soup *(see Chapter 5: The Joy of Soup).*

If you're out all day you'll probably have to roast your chicken on Sunday night, in which case, be careful not to overcook it or the chicken will be dry when you warm it up again. Once cooked, as soon as the chicken is cool enough to handle, carve the meat off and divide it into two casserole dishes, cover them with lids and store both lots in the fridge for Monday and Tuesday.

THE MONDAY ROAST:
Roast chicken
Potatoes
Parsnips
White cabbage
Peas
Carrots

METHOD
1. Peel the potatoes and par boil for a few minutes while you heat the fat in the oven *(see notes, page 99)*, then sprinkle with rosemary or a few sesame seeds if you feel like doing something different.
2. Cut the parsnips into small wedges and roast them alongside the potatoes.
3. Save ¼ of the cabbage to make coleslaw with at the end of the week if you like, otherwise cook the whole thing; there should plenty left over to make Bubble & Squeak on Wednesday. Store (cooked) leftover cabbage and carrots in the fridge, keeping them well covered to contain the smell.

TUESDAY:
CHICKEN & LEEK CASSEROLE
'Casserole' is a bit of an exaggeration for something as basic as this, but it looks and tastes a bit like a casserole, and I don't know what else to call it.

Remains of yesterday's chicken
1 tin condensed soup (chicken or mushroom)
Milk
2 leeks
Spinach
Oil & butter
Potatoes
Peas
Tarragon

METHOD
1. Peel potatoes (enough for tonight's dinner and tomorrow's Bubble
   & Squeak) and put them on to boil in a large saucepan of cold water.
2. Cut the chicken into chunks or small pieces, fry gently in a
   little oil and butter in another large saucepan, adding the
   tarragon or whatever herbs you want to use, if any.
3. Wash and finely chop the leeks and spinach and put them in the
   pan with the chicken; add the condensed soup, stir well and thin
   the soup down with a little milk until it reaches the consistency you
   want. Don't let the soup boil; cover the casserole with a lid and
   simmer gently until the potatoes are ready. (Transfer the casserole
   to an ovenproof dish and keep it warm in the oven if you like.)
4. Meanwhile, cook frozen peas in boiling water for a few
   minutes while you mash the potatoes, then serve.

WEDNESDAY:
BUBBLE, BANGERS & BEANS
Traditionally, Bubble & Squeak was made from leftover potatoes,
cabbage and onions mashed up together and fried in dripping,
but use whatever combination of leftover vegetables you like;
broccoli, peas and carrots, curly kale, Brussels sprouts; it doesn't
really matter. As long as you've got plenty of potato, anything goes.

METHOD

1. Cook sausages in the oven; it's less messy and you don't need any extra oil or fat (don't forget to prick the skins first).
2. Fry your Bubble in the biggest pan you've got and pre-heat the oil or lard until it's practically smoking. Alternatively, put it in a greased ovenproof dish, dotting the top all over with butter.
3. To save time and energy, warm the baked beans up in the oven, rather than use another saucepan or put them in the microwave – what's the point when you've got all that heat going to waste? Put the beans in a Pyrex dish on the bottom shelf, or on the oven floor, 10 minutes before the end of cooking time and give them a good stir when you take them out.

THURSDAY:

KEDGEREE *(see Chapter 3: Make Dinner, Not Excuses).*

FRIDAY:

CHEESE & SPINACH OMELETTE (WITH OVEN CHIPS)

Classic omelettes are made individually with three eggs (more cholesterol anyone?) by clever chefs who whisk and flip everything around in the pan until somehow they've produced a perfect, cigar-shaped omelette; firm on the outside, soft and still slightly runny on the inside. There's another, much easier way of making omelettes and you can get away with using only one egg per person, if that's all you've got, as long as there's plenty of filling.

If you've got the time and the inclination (it's Friday, remember) you can make coleslaw by finely shredding a bit of the leftover raw cabbage with thinly sliced carrot and onion, and adding a couple of spoonfuls of mayonnaise, or a mixture of mayonnaise and natural yoghurt. If you're having oven chips, put them in first and make the omelette – which only takes about ten minutes from start to finish – once the chips are almost done.

SERVES 4:
Eggs (4–6)
Spinach
Cheddar Cheese
Butter
Salt & pepper

METHOD

1. Grate the cheese, wash the spinach and tear it into small pieces, whisk the eggs with a fork and add a splash of cold water.
2. Warm the butter in a large frying pan, pour the eggs in, add the spinach and cheese and fluff the whole thing with a fork until it's all mixed up and the spinach is submerged.
3. Leave the omelette to set over a low heat for a few minutes, then take it off the heat and put it under the grill for another couple of minutes until the top of the omelette sets and rises and turns golden.

WEEK THREE

MONDAY:	Boiled Bacon & Roast Potatoes with Roasted Vegetables
TUESDAY:	Vegetable Tortilla
WEDNESDAY:	Pork Meatballs, Tagliatelle & Tomato Sauce
THURSDAY:	Stuffed Peppers
FRIDAY:	Pacific Pie

THE SHOPPING LIST:

Bacon joint	£3.29
Tuna	0.98
Cheese	£1.59

Chopped tomatoes	0.21
Plum tomatoes	0.13
Baked beans	0.17
Minced pork	£1.08
Sweetcorn	0.39
Spinach	£1.29
Mixed peppers	£2.58
Potatoes	£1.59
Savoy cabbage	0.58
Couscous	0.82
Mushrooms	£1.15
Butternut squash	£1.36
Tagliatelle	0.69
Eggs (12 free-range)	£1.75
Onions	0.16
Ready salted crisps (x 6)	0.85

£20.66

WEEK THREE: THE RECIPES

MONDAY:
BOILED BACON & ROAST POTATOES WITH ROASTED VEGETABLES
The bacon joint can be roasted or boiled (preferably ahead of time if you're out all day), then sliced up and re-heated at the bottom of the oven halfway through the cooking time of the roast vegetables. (If you've got more bacon than you want to use tonight, save some for tomorrow.)

Make more roasted vegetables than you need and keep the rest in the fridge for Tuesday's vegetable tortilla. The quantities below should be more than enough for four people with plenty to spare, especially if you're having roast potatoes and more green vegetables – otherwise, make more.

ROASTED VEGETABLES:

1 butternut squash

3 peppers: red, yellow, orange (preferably one of each)

4 –5 large, thin carrots

2 small onions (or 8 small shallots)

4 large mushrooms (or 6–8 small ones)

Sesame seeds, olive oil

GRAVY:

Gravy granules

Tomato puree

½ pint (250 ml) boiling water

METHOD

1. Peel potatoes first so you can par boil them on a low heat while you prepare the rest of the vegetables; roast them separately on a higher shelf and swap them over with the vegetables about halfway through.

2. Cut the butternut squash in half; peel the skin with a potato peeler, remove the pips and the foamy inner bit and cut into wedges.

3. Scrape the carrots and slice them diagonally; halve the peppers and cut them into strips; peel and slice the onion, or if you're using shallots, peel and cut them into halves or quarters; peel and cut the mushrooms into chunks.

4. Put the vegetables into a large ovenproof dish, drizzle with olive oil and sprinkle with sesame seeds.

5. In a measuring jug, mix 1 tablespoon of gravy granules with a little tomato puree, add boiling water up to the ½ pint (250 ml) mark and whisk with a fork. Pour the gravy over the bacon in an

ovenproof dish, cover with a lid or a piece of silver foil and put in the bottom of the oven until the roast potatoes and vegetables are done. (Or if you prefer, re-heat the bacon in the microwave.)

TUESDAY:
VEGETABLE TORTILLA
Not strictly a vegetable tortilla if you're adding leftover bacon, obviously...

SERVES 4–6:
2 tbsp plain flour
1 egg
½ pint (250 ml) milk
Remains of yesterday's roasted vegetables
(Leftover bacon)
Oil

METHOD
1. Pre-heat the oven on high, Gas Mark 7–8 (200–220°C) and warm a little oil in a very large ovenproof dish.
2. Make a thin pancake batter with the flour, egg and milk, mash the leftover roasted vegetables with a fork and beat the vegetable mash together with the batter to make a smooth paste.
3. If you've got leftover bacon, chop it into small pieces and put it into the hot oil first, then spread the veggie batter mix over the top to completely cover the bottom of the dish.
4. The tortilla cooks in about 20 minutes, so if you want baked beans and tinned plum tomatoes with it, put them in a covered casserole dish at the very bottom of the oven when you put the tortilla in; everything will be ready at the same time.

WEDNESDAY:

PORK MEATBALLS WITH TAGLIATELLE & TOMATO SAUCE
(see Chapter 3: Make Dinner, Not Excuses).

For an even quicker alternative to the DIY Pasta Sauce in
Chapter 3 make the easy tomato sauce below:

1 standard tin of chopped tomatoes

Tomato puree

Garlic puree

Spinach

1 onion or a few shallots

Herbs: basil, Italian herbs or parsley

Olive oil & butter

METHOD

1. Chop the onion or shallots; wash and tear spinach into
   small pieces.
2. Warm the oil and butter in a large shallow pan; add the onion,
   garlic and spinach and fry for a few minutes until the onion is soft.
3. Add the tinned tomatoes, turn the heat up and make it sizzle,
   then add herbs, tomato/garlic purees, stir well and simmer the
   sauce until the pasta is ready.

THURSDAY:

STUFFED PEPPERS *(see Chapter 3: Make Dinner, Not Excuses).*

FRIDAY:

PACIFIC PIE *(see Chapter 4: Quick Fixes).*

WEEK FOUR

MONDAY:	Liver, Bacon & Onions
TUESDAY:	Tomato & Red Lentil Soup
WEDNESDAY:	Salmon & Tomato Pasta Bake
THURSDAY:	Pork Ribs, Sausages & Rice
FRIDAY:	Bread Roll Pizzas

THE SHOPPING LIST:

Back bacon (x 2: Buy 1 Get 1 Free)	£ 2.59
Lamb's Liver	£ 1.02
Pork ribs	£ 3.39
Sausages (x 10: 82% pork)	£ 2.09
1 large tin of salmon (Alaskan)	£ 2.29
Lentils	0.69
Rice	0.55
Pasta	0.37
Soft bread rolls (very large x 12)	£ 1.50
Cheese	£ 1.29
Broccoli	0.65
Onions	0.39
Mushrooms	0.99
Spinach	0.99
Potatoes	£ 1.78
Fresh tomatoes	0.75
Cucumber	0.74
Tinned tomatoes (x 3)	£ 1.35
Pineapple rings	0.75
	£24.17

WEEK FOUR: THE RECIPES

MONDAY:
LIVER, BACON & ONIONS with mashed potatoes and green vegetables

SERVES 4 –6:
1–2 packets of lamb's liver
2 onions
1 packet of bacon (streaky or back)
½ pint (250 ml) lamb or beef stock
Tomato puree
Flour
Oil

METHOD
1. Peel the potatoes and put them on to simmer gently while you prepare the liver in the usual way, i.e. wash it well, removing any sinewy bits and coat in a little seasoned flour.
2. Warm some oil in a large pan and fry the liver for a couple of minutes before transferring to a casserole dish with a lid.
3. Fry the onions the way you like them and add the stock to the pan with a big spoonful of tomato puree; stir well, then pour the onion gravy into the casserole dish and put it in the middle of a moderate oven.
4. Roll up the bacon rashers and place on a baking tray on the top shelf of the oven.
5. When the bacon rolls are brown and crisp (about 20–25 minutes), slice thinly and scatter over the liver and onions, then serve with the mashed potatoes and green vegetables. (N.B. Make extra gravy if you think you need to.)

TUESDAY:

TOMATO & RED LENTIL SOUP *(see Chapter 5: The Joy of Soup)*.
Cheese on toast or bacon sandwiches are perfect with tomato soup.

WEDNESDAY:

SALMON & TOMATO PASTA BAKE
Needless to say, this can just as easily be made with tinned tuna
instead of salmon...

SERVES 4–6:
Tomato & red lentil soup
Pasta shapes
1 large tin of tuna
1 small tin of sweetcorn
Lemon juice
Black pepper
2 oz (50 g) grated cheese
1 packet of ready salted crisps, broken up in the bag

METHOD
1. If necessary, thin the soup with milk or tomato juice, or a
   combination of both.
2. Drain the tins of tuna and sweetcorn, empty into a large
   ovenproof dish, sprinkle with lemon juice and black pepper
   and mix with the tomato soup and uncooked pasta
   (approximately one generous handful per person).
3. Scatter the grated cheese and crushed crisps over the top and
   bake in a moderate oven, Gas Mark 4 (180°C) for about
   30–40 minutes.

THURSDAY:

PORK RIBS, SAUSAGES & RICE WITH SALAD

METHOD

1. First prick the sausages and put them in a hot oven, Gas Mark 6 (200°C).
2. After about 15 minutes, wash the rice and put in a pan of slightly salted boiling water, boil rapidly for a couple of minutes, then simmer very gently, checking after about 12 minutes to see if it's done.
3. Meanwhile, season the ribs, drizzle with a little olive oil and grill on high, turning at least once.
4. Make salad with tomatoes, spinach and cucumber from this week's shopping list, plus anything else you have and wish to include.
5. Strain the rice in a colander, rinse well with boiling water, and serve.

FRIDAY:

BREAD ROLL PIZZAS

These can be made with baguettes sliced lengthways, or readymade pizza bases if you prefer. *(See also Baked Potato Pizzas: Chapter 3: Make Dinner, Not Excuses)*.

Very large soft bread rolls, roughly 1 per person

Onions

Pineapple

Grated cheese

Leftover bacon and/or sausage

Spinach

Mushrooms

Tomatoes

Tomato puree or ketchup

Olive oil

METHOD

1. Slice the bread rolls in half and lightly toast the underside of each half under the grill while you warm some oil in a large pan.
2. Finely chop whatever you have to use for the toppings and fry everything except the pineapple for a few minutes, enough to soften the onion and brown the meat a little.
3. Spread the upper side of the bread rolls with tomato puree or ketchup, cover with the mixture, top with grated cheese and place under a hot grill for a few minutes, until the cheese has melted, browned and bubbled.

WEEK FIVE

MONDAY:	Corned Beef Hash
TUESDAY:	Fish Finger Pie
WEDNESDAY:	Spaghetti Bolognese
THURSDAY:	Curried Nut Roast & Rice
FRIDAY:	Gammon Steaks, Egg & Homemade Chips

THE SHOPPING LIST:

Minced beef (2 x 500 g packs)	£ 5.50
Corned beef (x 2 tins)	£ 2.38
Gammon steaks (x 4: large)	£ 5.88
Fish fingers (x 16)	£ 2.49
Eggs (12 free-range)	£ 2.35
Cheese	£ 2.49
Spaghetti	0.28
Rice	0.78
Bread	0.55
Monkey nuts (large 450 g bag)	£ 1.69
Tomato puree	0.32

Sweetcorn	0.63
Stock cubes (x 12)	0.76
Baked beans	0.47
Potatoes	£2.09
Spinach	£1.79
Mixed peppers	£1.38
Mushrooms	£1.49
Onions	0.55
Carrots	0.85
Asparagus	£1.99
Tomatoes	£1.89
Cucumber	0.75
	£39.43

WEEK FIVE: THE RECIPES

MONDAY:
CORNED BEEF HASH WITH BAKED BEANS

SERVES 4–6:
2 large tins of corned beef
2–3 lb (1.5k g) potatoes
2 large onions
Oil

METHOD
1. Peel and boil the potatoes until they're just done, then cut into cubes.
2. Warm the oil in a very large frying pan (or a large deep-sided pan to give you more room to manoeuvre) while you cut the

corned beef into chunks and slice the onions.

3. Fry the onions and potatoes in the hot oil, adding the corned beef once the onions are starting to brown.

4. Fry for a few more minutes until it looks good to you – and serve.

TUESDAY:
FISH FINGER PIE WITH POTATO WEDGES AND SWEETCORN
FISH FINGER PIE *(see Chapter 4, Quick Fixes)*.

POTATO WEDGES:
METHOD

1 Give the potatoes a quick wash with a nailbrush in a bowl of cold water; cut into wedges, place on a large ovenproof tray, drizzle with oil and bake in a hot oven, Gas Mark 6 (200°C) for 20–25 minutes.

2. Get the ingredients for the pies ready and grill the fish fingers after about 15 minutes, once the potatoes are halfway there.

WEDNESDAY:
SPAGHETTI BOLOGNESE
For young children, break the spaghetti into small pieces before putting it into the boiling water, or use small pasta shapes instead.

SERVES 4–6:
1 lb (500 g) (1 large pack) minced beef
1 onion
2 cloves of garlic
1 carrot, grated
Mushrooms
1 beef stock cube
1 standard tin of chopped tomatoes
Tomato puree
Oregano or Italian herbs

METHOD

1. Cook the meat in a large pan over a medium-high heat, turning it over occasionally with a wooden spoon while you prepare the vegetables.
2. Strain the meat to get rid of the fatty liquid, *(see notes, page 43),* add the finely chopped onion, mushrooms, grated carrot, crushed garlic, chopped tomatoes, tomato puree, stock cube and seasoning, and cook for a few more minutes.
3. Adjust the consistency of the bolognese with more tomato puree to make a richer sauce, or add a little beef stock if you want to thin it down.
4. Simmer gently for about 15 minutes while you cook the spaghetti; serve with grated cheddar cheese or parmesan.

THURSDAY:
CURRIED NUT ROAST
This nut roast is delicious hot or cold with salad and rice, or on its own with chutney or a yoghurt dressing. Buy monkey nuts if you can't get ready-shelled peanuts in the supermarket, or try a local shop; you'll find large bags of shelled nuts in any good Asian food store. *(For a nut-free alternative see Chapter 3: Make Dinner, Not Excuses.)*

SERVES 4–6:
½ lb (225 g) peanuts or cashew nuts
2 smallish peppers – red/orange and green
1 large onion
2 cloves of garlic
1 standard tin of chopped tomatoes
Breadcrumbs made with 4–5 slices of white bread
3 tsp curry powder
1 tsp cumin
Marjoram or mixed herbs

1 egg, beaten
Olive oil
Sunflower/corn oil

METHOD

1. Make the breadcrumbs in a blender or food processor then put them in a very large mixing bowl.
2. Blend the nuts for about 30 seconds and add them to the bowl.
3. Meanwhile, chop the onions and peppers and fry with the crushed garlic in a mixture of olive oil and sunflower, or corn oil, until the onion is crisp and golden.
4. Add the fried vegetables to the bowl with the chopped tomatoes, herbs, spices and the beaten egg and mix thoroughly – use a fork, it's easier – to bind everything together.
5. Press the mixture into a well greased, standard-sized loaf tin (long-strip-lined with greaseproof paper) and bake in a pre-heated oven, Gas Mark 6 (200°C) for about half an hour, until golden.
6. Cook the rice and make salad while the nut roast is in the oven, then cut into slices and serve.

FRIDAY:

GAMMON STEAKS, EGG & HOMEMADE CHIPS

There's no chip like a homemade chip and they're dead easy to make yourself, although you wouldn't think so to hear some celebrity chefs' advice on the subject, what with rinsing the potatoes under cold running water for 5 minutes (5 minutes! Doesn't anyone have a water meter?), flash-frying the chips in hot oil, then sprinkling them with this and that and finishing them off in the oven.

All you really need is good potatoes (Maris Pipers are ideal) and a very large saucepan about 2/3 full of hot oil – unless you've got a proper electric fryer (I haven't), in which case you'll know what to do.

1 gammon steak per person (although young children probably won't be able to eat more than half a steak)
Potatoes
Eggs
Asparagus

METHOD
1. Peel the potatoes, cut into chunky chips, roughly ½ inch (1.5 cm) thick and rinse well in cold running water for a mere 10 seconds.
2. Allow the chips to drain while you heat the oil, making sure you've got rid of every last drop of water with an old, clean tea towel or kitchen roll.
3. When a cube of stale bread dropped into the oil turns golden within seconds, the oil is hot enough.
4. If you have a chip basket big enough, use that, otherwise cook the chips loose, lowering them into the hot oil as carefully you can.
5. Cover with a lid and check them often; they should be ready in about 20 minutes.
6. Grill the gammon steaks about halfway through the chips' cooking time.
7. Remove the chips from the pan with a slotted spoon and drain them on plenty of kitchen roll on a large tray while you quickly fry an egg for each gammon steak and cook the asparagus spears in the microwave, according to the instructions on the packet.

Index

A

All-in-One Apple Cake 187
Apples
    All-in-One Apple Cake 187
    Baked Apples 147
    Poor Man's Apple Pie 149
    Sweet Apple and Apricot Pork 65
    Toffee 224
Apricot and Almond Muffins 192
Aubergine Lasagne 87

B

Bacon Cakes 110
Baked Apples 147
Baked Banana Custard 159
Baked Potato Pizzas 96
Banana Cake 186
Bean Soup, Spicy 126
Beef
    Beef and Cheese Crumble 51
    Beef Stroganoff 70
    Borsht 131
    Chilli Con Carne 47
    Hamburgers 49
    Rissoles 50
    Scotch Broth 134
    Spaghetti Bolognese 257
    Steak and Kidney Pudding 68
Biscuits, Easy Cheesy 171
Boiled Bacon 247
Borsht 131
Bran Loaf 183
Bread
    Garlic 212
    Hot Cross Buns 219
    Quick Brown 209
    Soda 210
Bread and Butter Pudding 151
Bread Pudding 188
Bread Roll Pizzas 254
Bubble, Bangers and Beans 244

C

Cakes
    All-in-One Apple 187
    Apricot and Almond Muffins 192
    Banana 186
    Bran Loaf 183
    Bread Pudding 188
    Carrot 182
    Caterpillar 199
    Chocolate Caramel 205
    Chocolate Rice Krispie 174
    Chocolate Yule Log 200
    Cornflake 175
    Fairy 175
    Flapjacks 189
    Ginger 185
    Gingerbread Men 177
    Honey, Lemon and Yoghurt 202
    Layer 201
    Muesli Muffins 194
    Plum 191
    Pumpkin Muffins 195
    Rock Buns 184
    Seed 190
    Sweetloaf 178
    Swiss Roll 196
    The Ultimate Chocolate 203
    Treacle Crunches 180
Carrot Cake 182
Caterpillar Cake 199
Celery Soup, Slug and 121
Cheesecake
    Cherry 143
    Cheshire Tart 145
    Lemon 144
Cheese and Courgette Scones 172
Cheese and Onion Tomatoes 97
Cheese and Spinach Omelette 245
Cherry Cheesecake 143
Cheshire Tart 145
Chicken
    Chicken in Cream and Mushroom
        Sauce 59
    Chicken Curry 54

Chicken Goujons 59
Chicken and Ham Pasta Bake 57
Chicken and Leek Casserole 243
Chicken Liver Pate 213
Chicken Liver Risotto 74
Chicken Nuggets 52
Chicken Soup 132
Chinese Chicken Stir Fry 241
Mexican Chicken 55
Roast Chicken 242
Sweet and Sour Chicken 58
Chilli Con Carne 47
Chips, Homemade 259
Chocolate Caramel Cakes 205
Chocolate Chip Cookies 180
Chocolate Mousse 153
Chocolate Rice Krispie Cakes 174
Chocolate Yule Log 200
Chutney 226
Cider Sausages 61
Cookies, Chocolate Chip 180
Cool Cucumber Soup 136
Corned Beef Hash 256
Corned Beef Hash, Instant 112
Cornflake Cakes 176
Cucumber Soup, Cool 136
Curry, Chicken 54
Curried Nut Roast 258

D
Devilled Kidneys 111
DIY Pasta Sauce 99

E
Easy Cheesy Biscuits 171

F
Fairy Cakes 175
Fastest-ever Fishcakes 116
Figgy Pudding 229
Fish
    Fastest-ever Fishcakes 116
    Fishcakes 81
    Fish Finger Pie 114
    Fish Pie 82
    Grilled Sardines 82
    Kedgeree 79
    Kipper Pate 214

Pacific Pie 107
Salmon and Tomato Pasta Bake 253
Smoked Mackerel Chowder 130
Smoked Salmon Tagliatelle 115
Things on Toast 117
Tuna Lasagne 77
Fishcakes 81
Fish Finger Pie 114
Fish Pie 82
Flapjacks 189
Fruit Fool 156
Fruit Jelly 159
Fudge 231

G
Gammon Steaks 259
Garlic Bread 212
Ginger Beer 222
Ginger Beer Pork 66
Gingerbread Men 177
Ginger Cake 185
Grapefruit Curd 228
Greek-style Pork 67
Grilled Sardines 82
Guacamole 214

H
Hamburgers 49
Hash Browns 218
Homemade Chips 259
Honeycomb 222
Honey, Lemon and Yoghurt Cake 202
Hot or Cold Leek and Potato Soup 137
Hot Cross Buns 219
Hummus 215

I
Ice-Cream, Raspberry 152
Instant Corned Beef Hash 112

J
Jam Tarts 173
Jelly, Fruit 159
Jimmy Young Trifle 150

K
Kebabs 72
Kedgeree 79

Kidneys, Devilled 111
Kipper Pate 214

L
Lancashire Hot Pot 71
Lamb
    Kebabs 72
    Lancashire Hot Pot 71
    Medallions of Lamb in Red Wine 73
    Moussaka 45
    Risssoles 50
    Scotch Broth 134
    Shepherd's Pie 44
Layer Cake 201
Leek and Potato Soup, Hot or Cold, 137
Lemon Cheesecake 144
Lentil Moussaka 88
Lentil and Vegetable Soup 125
Liver
    Chicken Liver Pate 213
    Chicken Liver Risotto 74
    Liver, Bacon and Onions 252
    Liver in Black Bean Sauce 75
    Spicy Liver and Pork Meatballs 76

M
Mayonnaise 216
Medallions of Lamb in Red Wine 73
Meringues, Strawberry 159
Mexican Chicken 55
Minestrone 128
Mixed Grill 76
More Noodles 109
Moussaka 45
    see also Lentil Moussaka 88
Muesli Muffins 194
Muffins
    Apricot and Almond 192
    Muesli 194
    Pumpkin 195
Mushrooms, Stuffed 84

N
Noodles 108
    see also More Noodles 109
Nut-free Nut Roast 92
Nut Roast, Curried 258
Nuts, Roasted 216

O
Omelette, Cheese and Spinach 245
One Step Pasta 112
Orange Cups 159
Orange Squash Soup 120

P
Pacific Pie 107
Pasta
    Aubergine Lasagne 87
    Chicken and Ham Pasta Bake 57
    One Step Pasta 112
    Salmon and Tomato Pasta Bake 253
    Smoked Salmon Tagliatelle 115
    Spaghetti Bolognese 257
    Tuna Lasagne 77
Pasta Sauce, DIY 99
Pate
    Chicken Liver 213
    Kipper 214
Peppers, Stuffed 83
Pizza 93
    see also Baked Potato Pizzas 96;
        Bread Roll Pizzas 254
Plum Cake 191
Poor Man's Apple Pie 149
Pork
    Ginger Beer Pork 66
    Greek-style Pork 67
    Pork in Plum Sauce 67
    Pork Ribs 253
    Rissoles 50
    Sausage Rolls 63
    Spicy Liver and Pork Meatballs 76
    Spicy Pork Meatballs 66
    Sweet Apple and Apricot Pork 65
Potato Salad 217
Potato Wedges 240
Prawn and Egg Pie 114
Prawns
    Prawn and Egg Pie 113
    Sweet and Spicy Prawns 78
Pumpkin Muffins 195

Q
Quick Brown Bread 209
Quorn Stir Fry 106

R
Raspberry Ice-Cream 152
Ratatouille 101
Rhubarb Crumble 148
Rice Salad 90
Rissoles 50
Roast Chicken 242
Roasted Nuts 216
Roast Vegetables 248
Rock Buns 184

S
Salmon and Tomato Pasta Bake 253
Sardines, Grilled 82
Sausages
    Bubble, Bangers and Beans 245
    Cider Sausages 61
    Toad in the Hole 60
Sausage Rolls 63
Scones, Cheese and Courgette 172
Scotch Broth 134
Seed Cake 190
Shepherd's Pie 44
Slug and Celery Soup 121
Smoked Mackerel Chowder 130
Smoked Salmon Tagliatelle 115
Soda Bread 210
Soft Fruit Spread 227
Soup
    Borsht 131
    Chicken 132
    Cool Cucumber 136
    Hot or Cold Leek and Potato 137
    Lentil and Vegetable 125
    Minestrone 128
    Orange Squash 120
    Slug and Celery 121
    Scotch Broth 134
    Smoked Mackerel Chowder 130
    Spicy Bean 126
    Stinging Nettle 123
    Sweet Potato 124
    Tomato and Red Lentil 127
    Watercress 122

Spaghetti Bolognese 257
Spicy Bean Soup 126
Spicy Liver and Pork Meatballs 76
Spicy Pork Meatballs 66
Spotted Dick 157
Steak and Kidney Pudding 68
Stinging Nettle Soup 123
Strawberry Meringues 159
Stroganoff, Beef 70
Stuffed Mushrooms 84
Stuffed Peppers 83
Sweet Apple and Apricot Pork 65
Sweetloaf 178
Sweet Potato Soup 124
Sweet and Sour Chicken 58
Sweet and Spicy Prawns 78
Swiss Roll 196

T
Things on Toast 117
The Ultimate Chocolate Cake 203
Tiramisu 155
Toad in the Hole 60
Toffee Apples 224
Tomato and Red Lentil Soup 127
Tomato Sauce 250
Tortilla, Vegetable 249
Treacle Crunches 180
Treacle Tart 154
Trifle, Jimmy Young 150
Tuna Lasagne 77

V
Veggie Burgers 85
Vegetable Soup, Lentil & 125
Vegetables, Roast 248
Vegetable Tortilla 249

W
Watercress Soup 122

Y
Yule Log, Chocolate 200